VACCINE DETOXIFICATION

C.J. Zingle

Dedicated to anyone who has ever been injured by a vaccine personally and for family and friends impacted by knowing someone who was or is vaccine injured.

The adversity faced is incomparable and the reward will be your strength for having gone through this adversity.

God's strongest warriors are given the hardest battles to overcome.

You are stronger than you know!

CONTENTS

DISCLAIMER

THIS INFORMATION IS INTENDED FOR EDUCATIONAL AND INFORMATIONAL PURPOSES ONLY and only summarizes a host of reference materials. It is not meant to replace qualified medical care and does not include all the information that may be of relevance for each herb or supplement. Every effort has been made to ensure that the information contained in this book is complete and accurate. The statements made in this book have not been evaluated by the U.S. Food and Drug Administration (FDA). The products mentioned in this book are not intended to treat, diagnose, cure, or prevent any disease or illness. The information provided in this book is not a substitute for a consultation with your own physician, and should not be construed as individual medical advice. Although this book contains information relating to health care, the information is not intended as medical advice and is not intended to replace a person-to-person relationship with a qualified healthcare professional. If you know or suspect you have a health problem, it is recommended that you first seek the advice of a physician before trying out any medical program or treatment. All efforts have been made to assure the accuracy of the information contained in this book at the time of publication.

The author disclaims any liability for any medical outcomes that may occur as a result of applying the methods suggested in this book.

PREFACE

This is an updated protocol to detox those who have been injected with the jab and the same protocol is useful to protect those concerned with the spike protein shedding coming off those who have been injected. If you know someone who has been injected and requires help, please provide them with this protocol.

It is important to detox with the below protocols as soon as possible. The longer you wait, the more time the vaccine has to incubate and react within the body and the more likely there is to be health damages. I have personally used all of the products below along with the protocols I have outlined. I have also received great feedback from everyone I have shared this with so far. There have been many people who have reached out to me in regret of receiving the vaccine and it is important to remember you are not alone and to keep faith and pray for healing and resolution.

The protocols below will also be very helpful for anyone who has suffered from a vaccine injury in the past. Unbeknownst to many, there are many people who suffer from vaccine injury and a lot of these injuries go undiagnosed and/or mistreated. Many Chronic diseases, illnesses, neurological disorders, cancers, etc. are triggered by vaccines. There is a reason they are considered a "mystery" and "incurable".

Cancer and disease are billion-dollar industries. There is no money in "The Cure" and the pharmaceutical industry knows this.

"There is no money in healthy people."

Blog Post - Click Here:
Over 1,000 Scientific Studies That Prove The COVID-19 Vaccines Are Dangerous (zinglepathy.com)

IF YOU BELIEVE
VACCINES SAVE LIVES
I HAVE 40 QUESTIONS FOR YOU

1. Name five vaccine ingredients
2. What is MRC-5?
3. What is WI-38?
4. What is vaccine court?
5. What is the National Vaccine Injury Compensation Program?
6. What is the 1986 National Childhood Vaccine Injury Act?
7. How has the CDC schedule changed since 1986?
8. How much money has been paid out by vaccine injury court?
9. How many doses of how many vaccines are in the CDC schedule between birth and age 16 (70 in US)?
10. Do vaccines contain aborted fetal tissue? If so, which vaccines? How many aborted babies were needed before they found one with the virus necessary to create the vaccine?
11. Do any vaccines contain dog, monkey, pig, and human DNA?
12. What is an adjuvant?
13. What is an antigen?
14. Which arm of the immune system do vaccines stimulate?
15. Which arms of the immune system do natural diseases stimulate?
16. What is transverse myelitis?
17. What is encephalopathy?
18. What is the rate of autism in 2017, what was it in 2000? What was it in 1990?
19. What is glyphosate and is it in vaccines?
20. If your child is injured, who will take physical, emotional, and financial responsibility?
21. What was the Supreme Court's statement on vaccines in 2011?
22. Can you provide a study showing vaccinated vs. unvaccinated health outcomes?
23. Can you show me a safety study proving it is safe to inject multiple vaccines?
24. What is shedding?
25. Do vaccines shed? Which vaccines can shed for up to six weeks?
26. Which vaccines are live virus vaccines?
27. What is the VICP?
28. What is SV40?
29. What is MTHFR (Methylenetetrahydrofolate Reductase)?
30. What is an acceptable amount of aluminum to ingest per day and how much is injected via the Hep B vaccine on day one of life?
31. Can someone who was vaccinated for pertussis still spread pertussis after being exposed to it? If so, for how long?
32. What is the death rate from measles in the US from 2005-2015? From the MMR vaccine in same time frame?
33. What does attenuated mean?
34. Where can I find information about vaccines?
35. Are there vaccine consent forms?
36. Can the vial stopper cause allergic reaction?
37. Can there be serious reactions to vaccines?
38. What is NVIC?
39. Is there any compensation for physicians who have a certain percentage of their patients vaccinated?
40. What's the difference between natural formaldehyde and synthetic? Which one is in vaccines?

RESEARCH.

FOR 1-ON-1 CONSULTATION & GUIDANCE

For 1-on-1 Consultation & Guidance With Me - Please Click Here:

https://form.jotform.com/Zinglepathy_Rx/detox-order-form

VACCINE INJURIES CONNECTED TO MAJOR HEALTH ILLNESSES

Frequently reported Neurological adverse effects

Adverse effect		Vaccines
Demyelination disease	Multiple sclerosis (MS)	Hepatitis B vaccine [50]
	Acute disseminated encephalomyelitis (ADEM)	Human papillomavirus vaccine [51]
	Transverse myelitis	Influenza vaccine
	Optic neuritis	Rabies vaccine [52]
		Yellow fever vaccine [53]
Guillain-Barré syndrome (GBS)		Influenza vaccine [54]
		Oral polio vaccine
		Tetanus vaccines [55]
Encephalopathy		Whole-cell pertussis vaccine [56]
		Influenza Vaccine
Seizure		Diphtheria, tetanus toxoids and whole-cell pertussis vaccine (DTP)
		Measles, mumps, and rubella vaccine (MMR) [9]
Autism		MMR [57], [a]

[a]The original manuscript had been withdrawn.

AUTOIMMUNE DISEASE

idiopathic thrombocytopenic purpura
Arthralgia/Arthritis including rheumatoid arthritis
Neurologic disease- related to yellow fever
Dermatomyositis
Takayasu's arteritis
Optic neuritis
Guillain Barre Syndrome (GBS)
Myelitis
Multiple Sclerosis
Systemic lupus erythematosus (SLE)
Antiphospholipid syndrome (APS)
Myopathy/Myositis
Acute disseminated encephalomyelitis
Transverse Myelitis
Pancreatitis
Postural Orthostatic tachycardia syndrome (POT)
Primary Ovarian Failure (POF)
Autoimmune hepatitis
Vasculitis
Henoch-Schonlein purpura (HSP)
Bullous Pemphigiod
Narcolepsy
Celliac disease
Polymyalgia rheumatica
Fibromyalgia/Chronic Fatigue syndrome

@cjzingle

VACCINE

Measles, mumps, nubela (MMR)
Yellow fever
Bacillus Calmette-Guerin (BCG)
Hepatitis B virus (HBV)
Human Papilloma Virus (HPV)
Influenza
Meningococcal
Pneumococcal
Diphtheria-Tetanus-Pertussis (dTP)
Varicella
Small Pox
Arthrex
H1N1 Influenza
Rotavirus

3

Vaccine Injury is nothing new... it's just rarely talked about...

Vaccine injuries are more common than most people know.

This post will include the following sections below:

- Vaccination as Contamination
- Aseptic Meningitis and the MMR
- Vaccinations and Leukemia/Lymphomas
- Vaccines and Chromosome Changes Leading to Mutations
- Vaccines and Autoimmunity
- Vaccinations and Diabetes
- Other Articles Linking Diabetes to Vaccines
- Vaccines and Nervous System Changes
- Vaccines and Demyelination
- Vaccinations and Seizures
- Vaccines and Brain Swelling
- Vaccines and Neurological Damage
- Vaccinations and Unexplained Diseases
- Vaccines and Metabolism
- Vaccines and Skin Disorders
- The Polio Vaccine and Cancer
- Vaccinations and Autism
- Resolving and Reversing Vaccine Injury

VACCINES DOSES for U.S. CHILDREN

1962	1983	2018	
TOTAL DOSES: 5	**TOTAL DOSES: 24**	**TOTAL DOSES: 72**	
Polio	DTP (2 months)	Influenza (pregnancy)	Influenza (18 months)
Smallpox	OPV (2 months)	DTaP (pregnancy)	Hep A (18 months)
DTP	DTP (4 months)	Hep B (birth)	Influenza (30 months)
	OPV (4 months)	Hep B (2 months)	Influenza (42 months)
	DTP (6 months)	Rotavirus (2 months)	DTaP (4 years)
	MMR (15 months)	DTaP (2 months)	IPV (4 years)
	DTP (18 months)	HIB (2 months)	MMR (4 years)
	OPV (18 months)	PCV (2 months)	Varicella (4 years)
	DTP (4 years)	IPV (2 months)	Influenza (5 years)
	OPV (4 years)	Rotavirus (4 months)	Influenza (6 years)
	Td (15 years)	DTaP (4 months)	Influenza (7 years)
		HIB (4 months)	Influenza (8 years)
		PCV (4 months)	Influenza (9 years)
		IPV (4 months)	HPV (9 years)
		Hep B (6 months)	Influenza (10 years)
		Rotavirus (6 months)	HPV (10 years)
		DTaP (6 months)	Influenza (11 years)
		HIB (6 months)	HPV (11 years)
		PCV (6 months)	DTaP (12 years)
		IPV (6 months)	Influenza (12 years)
		Influenza (6 months)	Meningococcal (12 years)
		Influenza (7 months)	Influenza (13 years)
		HIB (12 months)	Influenza (14 years)
		PCV (12 months)	Influenza (15 years)
		MMR (12 months)	Influenza (16 years)
		Varicella (12 months)	Meningococcal (16 years)
		Hep A (12 months)	Influenza (17 years)
		DTaP (18 months)	Influenza (18 years)

*In 1986, pharmaceutical companies producing vaccines were given full federal protection from lawsuits resulting from vaccine injury or death via the Childhood Vaccine Injury Act passed by Congress. If vaccines are so safe, why did they need a law to protect from liability?

After this law, vaccines became HIGHLY profitable. There are almost 300 vaccines in development, and mandatory vaccine laws for children — and ADULTS — being pushed in most states.

The US gives 2-3x more vaccines to children than most developed countries, yet we have skyrocketing rates of childhood issues that are NOT seen in other countries. Things like asthma, childhood diabetes, food allergies, childhood leukemia, developmental delays, tics, ADHD, autism, lupus, arthritis, eczema, epilepsy, Alzheimers, brain damage, etc… It's NOT a coincidence.

Vaccines contain toxic chemicals that do NOT belong in our bodies, such as aluminum (known to cause brain and developmental damage even in small doses), polysorbate 80, MSG and formaldehyde (known to cause cancer in humans).

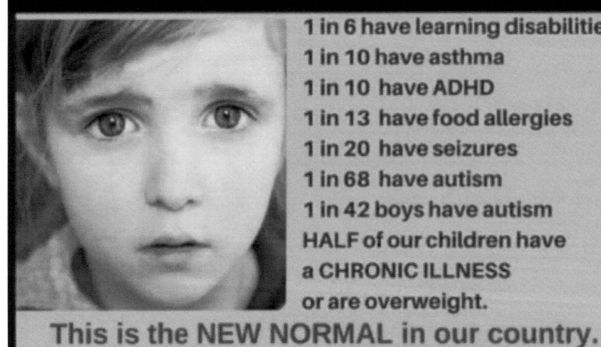

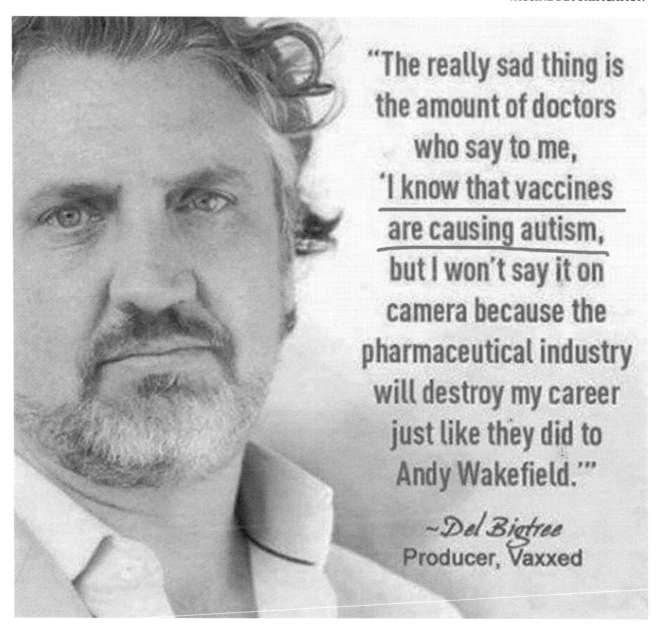

"The really sad thing is the amount of doctors who say to me, 'I know that vaccines are causing autism, but I won't say it on camera because the pharmaceutical industry will destroy my career just like they did to Andy Wakefield.'"

~Del Bigtree
Producer, Vaxxed

For More Information On Vaccine Injury Studies: Maybe It's 'Genetics' OR Maybe It's a VACCINE INJURY - A Compilation Of Historical Vaccine Injury Studies (zinglepathy.com)

Blog Post - Click Here:
Over 1,000 Scientific Studies That Prove The COVID-19 Vaccines Are Dangerous (zinglepathy.com)

COVID-19 VACCINE INSERTS & WARNINGS

FDA NEWS RELEASE

Coronavirus (COVID-19) Update: June 25, 2021

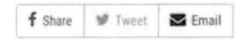

For Immediate Release:

June 25, 2021

The U.S. Food and Drug Administration (FDA) continued to take action in the ongoing response to the COVID-19 pandemic:

- Today, the FDA is announcing revisions to the patient and provider fact sheets for the Moderna and Pfizer-BioNTech COVID-19 vaccines regarding the suggested increased risks of myocarditis (inflammation of the heart muscle) and pericarditis (inflammation of the tissue surrounding the heart) following vaccination. For each vaccine, the Fact Sheet for Healthcare Providers Administering Vaccine (Vaccination Providers) has been revised to include a warning about myocarditis and pericarditis and the Fact Sheet for Recipients and Caregivers has been revised to include information about myocarditis and pericarditis. This update

Serious Adverse Events

Pfizer-BioNTech - Drug Insert

In Study 2, among participants 16 through 55 years of age who had received at least 1 dose of vaccine or placebo (COMIRNATY =12,995; placebo = 13,026), serious adverse events from Dose 1 up to the participant unblinding date in ongoing follow-up were reported by 103 (0.8%) COMIRNATY recipients and 117 (0.9%) placebo recipients. In a similar analysis, in participants 56 years of age and older (COMIRNATY = 8,931; placebo = 8,895), serious adverse events were reported by 165 (1.8%) COMIRNATY recipients and 151 (1.7%) placebo recipients who received at least 1 dose of COMIRNATY or placebo, respectively. In these analyses, 58.2% of study participants had at least 4 months of follow-up after Dose 2. Among participants with confirmed stable HIV infection serious adverse events from Dose 1 up to the participant unblinding date in ongoing follow-up were reported by 2 (2%) COMIRNATY recipients and 2 (2%) placebo recipients.

In the analysis of blinded, placebo-controlled follow-up, there were no notable patterns between treatment groups for specific categories of serious adverse events (including neurologic, neuro-inflammatory, and thrombotic events) that would suggest a causal relationship to COMIRNATY. In the analysis of unblinded follow-up, there were no notable patterns of specific categories of serious adverse events that would suggest a causal relationship to COMIRNATY.

6.2   Postmarketing Experience

The following adverse reactions have been identified during postmarketing use of COMIRNATY, including under Emergency Use Authorization. Because these reactions are reported voluntarily from a population of uncertain size, it is not always possible to reliably estimate their frequency or establish a causal relationship to vaccine exposure.

Cardiac Disorders: myocarditis, pericarditis
Gastrointestinal Disorders: diarrhea, vomiting
Immune System Disorders: severe allergic reactions, including anaphylaxis, and other hypersensitivity reactions (e.g., rash, pruritus, urticaria, angioedema)
Musculoskeletal and Connective Tissue Disorders: pain in extremity (arm)

<u>Unsolicited Adverse Events</u>

Pfizer-BioNTech - Drug Insert

Overall, 11,253 (51.1%) participants in the COMIRNATY group and 11,316 (51.4%) participants in the placebo group had follow-up time between ≥4 months to <6 months after Dose 2 in the blinded placebo-controlled follow-up period with an additional 1,778 (8.1%) and 1,304 (5.9%) with ≥6 months of blinded follow-up time in the COMIRNATY and placebo groups, respectively.

A total of 12,006 (54.5%) participants originally randomized to COMIRNATY had ≥6 months total (blinded and unblinded) follow-up after Dose 2.

In an analysis of all unsolicited adverse events reported following any dose, through 1 month after Dose 2, in participants 16 years of age and older (N=43,847; 21,926 COMIRNATY group vs. 21,921 placebo group), those assessed as adverse reactions not already captured by solicited local and systemic reactions were nausea (274 vs. 87), malaise (130 vs. 22), lymphadenopathy (83 vs. 7), asthenia (76 vs. 25), decreased appetite (39 vs. 9), hyperhidrosis (31 vs. 9), lethargy (25 vs. 6), and night sweats (17 vs. 3).

In analyses of all unsolicited adverse events in Study 2 from Dose 1 up to the participant unblinding date, 58.2% of study participants had at least 4 months of follow-up after Dose 2. Among participants 16 through 55 years of age who received at least 1 dose of study vaccine, 12,995 of whom received COMIRNATY and 13,026 of whom received placebo, unsolicited adverse events were reported by 4,396 (33.8%) participants in the COMIRNATY group and 2,136 (16.4%) participants in the placebo group. In a similar analysis in participants 56 years of age and older that included 8,931 COMIRNATY recipients and 8,895 placebo recipients, unsolicited adverse events were reported by 2,551 (28.6%) participants in the COMIRNATY group and 1,432 (16.1%) participants in the placebo group. Among participants with confirmed stable HIV infection that included 100 COMIRNATY recipients and 100 placebo recipients, unsolicited adverse events were reported by 29 (29%) participants in the COMIRNATY group and 15 (15%) participants in the placebo group. The higher frequency of reported unsolicited adverse events among COMIRNATY recipients compared to placebo recipients was primarily attributed to events that are consistent with adverse reactions solicited among participants in the reactogenicity subset (Table 3 and Table 4).

Throughout the placebo-controlled safety follow-up period, Bell's palsy (facial paralysis) was reported by 4 participants in the COMIRNATY group and 2 participants in the placebo group. Onset of facial paralysis was Day 37 after Dose 1 (participant did not receive Dose 2) and Days 3, 9, and 48 after Dose 2. In the placebo group the onset of facial paralysis was Day 32 and Day 102. Currently available information is insufficient to determine a causal relationship with the vaccine. In the analysis of blinded, placebo-controlled follow-up, there

14

were no other notable patterns or numerical imbalances between treatment groups for specific categories of non-serious adverse events (including other neurologic or neuro-inflammatory, and thrombotic events) that would suggest a causal relationship to COMIRNATY. In the analysis of unblinded follow-up, there were no notable patterns of specific categories of non-serious adverse events that would suggest a causal relationship to COMIRNATY.

5 WARNINGS AND PRECAUTIONS

Moderna Vaccine - Drug Insert

5.1 Management of Acute Allergic Reactions

Appropriate medical treatment to manage immediate allergic reactions must be immediately available in the event an acute anaphylactic reaction occurs following administration of SPIKEVAX.

5.2 Myocarditis and Pericarditis

Postmarketing data demonstrate increased risks of myocarditis and pericarditis, particularly within 7 days following the second dose. The observed risk is higher among males under 40 years of age than among females and older males. The observed risk is highest in males 18 through 24 years of age. Although some cases required intensive care support, available data from short-term follow-up suggest that most individuals have had resolution of symptoms with conservative management. Information is not yet available about potential long-term sequelae. The CDC has published considerations related to myocarditis and pericarditis after vaccination,

3

including for vaccination of individuals with a history of myocarditis or pericarditis (https://www.cdc.gov/vaccines/covid-19/clinical-considerations/myocarditis.html).

FDA warnings: In July, the FDA attached a warning to the Johnson & Johnson vaccine after rare cases of the neurological disorder Guillain-Barré syndrome were reported in a small number of vaccination recipients. Most of the cases occurred within 42 days after vaccination.

FDA WARNING: Johnson & Johnson Vaccine In April, the FDA added a warning label after ending a pause on the vaccine it had recommended "out of an abundance of caution" over an uncommon, but potentially serious, blood clotting disorder that occurred in a small number of recipients.

In December, the FDA updated its fact sheet on the shot to include information about the rare but serious blood clotting disorder called thrombosis with thrombocytopenia syndrome (TTS) associated with the vaccine. The agency still says the risks of the virus are greater than the risks of the J&J vaccine.

[2021]

WARNINGS

Management of Acute Allergic Reactions

Appropriate medical treatment to manage immediate allergic reactions must be immediately available in the event an acute anaphylactic reaction occurs following administration of the Janssen COVID-19 Vaccine.

Monitor Janssen COVID-19 Vaccine recipients for the occurrence of immediate adverse reactions according to the Centers for Disease Control and Prevention guidelines (https://www.cdc.gov/vaccines/covid-19/clinical-considerations/managing-anaphylaxis.html).

Thrombosis with Thrombocytopenia Syndrome (TTS)

Reports to the Vaccine Adverse Events Reporting System (VAERS), a passive surveillance system, provide evidence for an increased risk of thrombosis with thrombocytopenia syndrome (TTS) with onset of symptoms approximately one to two weeks after administration of the Janssen COVID-19 Vaccine. An analysis of VAERS reports of TTS following the receipt of the Janssen COVID-19 Vaccine used the following case definition:

- a thrombosis in an unusual location for a thrombus (i.e., cerebral vein, visceral artery or vein, extremity artery, central artery or vein) and new-onset thrombocytopenia (i.e., platelet count <150,000/µL) occurring any time after vaccination;
  or
- new-onset thrombocytopenia (i.e., platelet count <150,000/µL), thrombosis in an extremity vein or pulmonary artery in the absence of thrombosis at an unusual location, and a positive anti-PF4 antibody ELISA test or functional Heparin-Induced Thrombocytopenia (HIT) platelet test occurring any time after vaccination.

Cases of TTS following administration of the Janssen COVID-19 Vaccine have been reported in males and females, in a wide age range of individuals 18 years and older, with the highest reporting rate (approximately 1 case per 100,000 doses administered) in females ages 30-49 years; overall, approximately 15% of TTS cases have been fatal. Currently available evidence supports a causal relationship between TTS and the Janssen COVID-19 Vaccine. The clinical course of these events shares features with autoimmune heparin-induced thrombocytopenia. In individuals with suspected TTS following administration of the Janssen COVID-19 Vaccine, the use of heparin may be harmful and alternative treatments may be needed. Consultation with hematology specialists is strongly recommended. The American Society of Hematology has published considerations relevant to the diagnosis and treatment of TTS following administration of the Janssen COVID-19 Vaccine (*https://www.hematology.org/covid-19/vaccine-induced-immune-thrombotic-thrombocytopenia*). (*see Full EUA Prescribing Information*).

Immune Thrombocytopenia (ITP)

Reports of adverse events following use of the Janssen COVID-19 Vaccine under emergency use authorization suggest an increased risk of immune thrombocytopenia (ITP) during the 42 days following vaccination. Individuals with a history of ITP should discuss with their healthcare

Revised: JAN/31/2022

Johnson & Johnson - Drug Insert

provider the risk of ITP and the potential need for platelet monitoring following vaccination with the Janssen COVID-19 Vaccine.

Guillain-Barré Syndrome

Reports of adverse events following use of the Janssen COVID-19 Vaccine under emergency use authorization suggest an increased risk of Guillain-Barré syndrome during the 42 days following vaccination.

Altered Immunocompetence

Immunocompromised persons, including individuals receiving immunosuppressant therapy, may have a diminished immune response to the Janssen COVID-19 Vaccine.

Syncope

Syncope (fainting) may occur in association with administration of injectable vaccines. Procedures should be in place to avoid injury from fainting.

Limitations of Vaccine Effectiveness

The Janssen COVID-19 Vaccine may not protect all vaccinated individuals.

ADVERSE REACTIONS

Johnson & Johnson - Drug Insert

Adverse Reactions in Clinical Trials

Adverse reactions reported in a clinical trial following administration of the Janssen COVID-19 Vaccine include injection site pain, headache, fatigue, myalgia, nausea, fever, injection site erythema and injection site swelling. In clinical studies, severe allergic reactions, including anaphylaxis, have been reported following administration of the Janssen COVID-19 Vaccine *(see Full EUA Prescribing Information)*.

Adverse Reactions Identified during Post Authorization Use

Anaphylaxis and other severe allergic reactions, thrombosis with thrombocytopenia, Guillain-Barré syndrome, and capillary leak syndrome have been reported following administration of the Janssen COVID-19 Vaccine during mass vaccination outside of clinical trials.

Additional adverse reactions, some of which may be serious, may become apparent with more widespread use of the Janssen COVID-19 Vaccine.

USE WITH OTHER VACCINES

There is no information on the co-administration of the Janssen COVID-19 Vaccine with other vaccines.

INFORMATION TO PROVIDE TO VACCINE RECIPIENTS/CAREGIVERS

As the vaccination provider, you must communicate to the recipient or their caregiver, information consistent with the "Fact Sheet for Recipients and Caregivers" (and provide a copy or direct the

Revised: JAN/31/2022

Vaccine Insert Source Links:

Moderna Insert: Moderna COVID-19 Vaccine Health Care Provider Fact Sheet (fda.gov)

Pfizer-BioNTech: Package Insert Comrinaty (purple cap) (fda.gov)

Janssen (J&J): Janssen COVID-19 Vaccine EUA Fact Sheet for Recipients and Caregivers (fda.gov)

TABLE 3. Events* reported to the Vaccine Adverse Event Reporting System for persons aged ≥12 years[†] after receipt of a bivalent Pfizer-BioNTech or Moderna COVID-19 vaccine booster dose — United States, August 31–October 23, 2022

Adverse events	Vaccine, no. reporting (%)		
	Pfizer-BioNTech	Moderna	Total[§]
Total	2,928	2,615	5,542
Vaccination errors[¶]	877 (30.0)	1,037 (39.7)	1,913 (34.5)
Error without adverse health event	717 (81.8)	972 (93.7)	1,688 (88.2)
Error with adverse health event**	160 (18.2)	65 (6.3)	225 (11.8)
Error with nonserious health event[††]	157 (17.9)	61 (5.9)	218 (11.4)
Error with serious health event	3 (0.3)	4 (0.4)	7 (0.4)
Nonserious reports[§§,¶¶]	2,762 (94.3)	2,530 (96.8)	5,291 (95.5)
Headache	343 (12.4)	285 (11.3)	628 (11.9)
Fatigue	318 (11.5)	257 (10.2)	575 (10.9)
Fever	299 (10.8)	262 (10.4)	561 (10.6)
Pain	293 (10.6)	231 (9.1)	524 (9.9)
Chills	254 (9.2)	205 (8.1)	459 (8.7)
Pain in extremity	209 (7.8)	167 (6.6)	376 (7.1)
Nausea	213 (7.7)	144 (5.7)	357 (6.8)
Dizziness	212 (7.7)	135 (5.3)	347 (6.6)
Injection site pain	138 (5.0)	121 (4.8)	259 (4.9)
COVID-19	169 (6.1)	89 (3.5)	258 (4.9)
Serious reports***,[†††]	166 (5.7)	85 (3.3)	251 (4.5)
Allergic reaction/Anaphylaxis	6	2	8
Appendicitis	4	1	5
Arrythmia	8	5	13
Atrial fibrillation	5	4	9
Atrioventricular node block, second or third degree	2	0	2
Supraventricular tachycardia	0	1	1
Other	1	0	1
COVID-19	14	6	20
Death[§§§]	27	9	36
Dyspnea	4	1	5
Fall	1	6	7
Guillain-Barré syndrome	2	0	2
Hypertension, acute	7	3	10
Pericarditis[¶¶¶]	1	3	4
Pneumonia	6	1	7
Seizure	6	0	6
Thrombotic event	20	11	31
Stroke or transient ischemic attack	12	5	17
Pulmonary embolism	5	5	10
Other	3	1	4
Chest pain, not otherwise specified	9	3	12
Myocardial infarction	5	3	8
Myocarditis****	3	2	5

Abbreviations: MedDRA PT = Medical Dictionary for Regulatory Activities preferred term; VAERS = Vaccine Adverse Event Reporting System.

* Signs and symptoms in VAERS reports are assigned MedDRA PTs by VAERS staff members. Each VAERS report might be assigned more than one MedDRA PT, which can include normal diagnostic findings. A MedDRA PT does not indicate a medically confirmed diagnosis.

[†] On August 31, 2022, the Food and Drug Administration authorized bivalent formulations of Moderna and Pfizer-BioNTech COVID-19 vaccines for use as a single booster dose ≥2 months after completing primary or booster vaccination, Pfizer-BioNTech for persons aged ≥12 years and Moderna for adults aged ≥18 years.

[§] One report was for a person who received both Moderna and Pfizer-BioNTech bivalent booster doses at the same visit and did not experience an adverse health event.

[¶] Vaccine administration or handling errors.

** The most common MedDRA PTs among reports of vaccination error included incorrect product formulation administered, incorrect dose administered, underdose, and wrong product administered.

[††] Adverse health events coded for reports with nonserious vaccination errors included arthralgia, headache, injection site erythema, injection site swelling, fever, pain, and pain in extremity.

[§§] Excluding vaccination error MedDRA PTs.

[¶¶] Includes the top 10 most frequently coded MedDRA PTs among nonserious reports.

*** VAERS reports are classified as serious if any of the following are reported: hospitalization, prolongation of hospitalization, life-threatening illness, permanent disability, congenital anomaly or birth defect, or death. Serious reports to VAERS were reviewed by CDC physicians to form preliminary clinical impressions. https://www.meddra.org/how-to-use/basics/hierarchy

[†††] Because of the small number of serious reports, percentages are not provided for serious report events. Other clinical impressions included acute pancreatitis, acute respiratory failure, aneurysm, arm pain, arthralgia, aseptic meningitis, bilateral pleural effusion, cellulitis, chronic anemia, compression fracture, confusion, contact dermatitis, costochondritis, erythema nodosum, fever, glaucoma, hearing loss, leukocytoplastic vasculitis, lower extremity weakness, lymphadenopathy, migraine, myalgia, pancreatitis, pericardial and pleural effusions, pericardial tamponade, pylephlebitis, rhabdomyolysis, unspecified bradycardia, unspecified tachycardia, transverse myelitis, vertigo, and vision loss.

[§§§] For reports of death, cause of death was available for four reports: cardiac arrest, dementia, metastatic prostate cancer, and myocardial infarction.

[¶¶¶] All four reports of pericarditis have been verified by medical record review.

**** Three of the five reports of myocarditis have been verified by medical record review.

(Source: Safety Monitoring of Bivalent COVID-19 mRNA Vaccine Booster Doses Among Persons Aged ≥12 Years — United States, August 31–October 23, 2022 (cdc.gov))

	Both mRNA vaccines (n=340 522)*	BNT162b2 vaccine (n=164 669)	mRNA-1273 vaccine (n=175 816)
Category			
Non-serious	313 499 (92·1%)	150 486 (91·4%)	162 977 (92·7%)
Serious, including death	27 023 (7·9%)	14 183 (8·6%)	12 839 (7·3%)
Serious, excluding death	22 527 (6·6%)	12 078 (7·3%)	10 448 (5·9%)
Death	4496 (1·3%)	2105 (1·3%)	2391 (1·4%)
Sex			
Female	246 085 (72·3%)	116 587 (70·8%)	129 475 (73·6%)
Male	88 311 (25·9%)	45 157 (27·4%)	43 140 (24·5%)
Unknown	6126 (1·8%)	2925 (1·8%)	3201 (1·8%)
Age, years			
16–17	6874 (2·0%)	3283 (2·0%)	3591 (2·0%)
18–49	154 171 (45·3%)	76 385 (46·4%)	77 773 (44·2%)
50–64	84 949 (24·9%)	40 367 (24·5%)	44 572 (25·4%)
65–74	49 755 (14·6%)	20 048 (12·2%)	29 702 (16·9%)
75–84	21 418 (6·3%)	9021 (5·5%)	12 392 (7·1%)
≥85	7595 (2·2%)	3564 (2·2%)	4027 (2·3%)
Unknown	15 760 (4·6%)	12 001 (7·3%)	3759 (2·1%)
Race or ethnicity†			
Hispanic or Latino	23 480 (6·9%)	11 217 (6·8%)	12 260 (7·0%)
Non-Hispanic			
White	169 877 (49·9%)	73 398 (44·6%)	96 469 (54·9%)
Black	10 446 (3·1%)	5104 (3·1%)	5342 (3·0%)
Asian	10 172 (3·0%)	5038 (3·1%)	5131 (2·9%)
American Indian or Alaska Native	1414 (0·4%)	615 (0·4%)	799 (0·5%)
Native Hawaiian or other Pacific Islander	441 (0·1%)	209 (0·1%)	232 (0·1%)
Multiple races	3542 (1·0%)	1578 (1·0%)	1964 (1·1%)
Other race	1684 (0·5%)	808 (0·5%)	876 (0·5%)
Unknown race	2593 (0·8%)	1422 (0·9%)	1171 (0·7%)
Unknown ethnicity			
White	28 787 (8·5%)	15 497 (9·4%)	13 289 (7·6%)
Black	4189 (1·2%)	2524 (1·5%)	1662 (1·0%)
Asian	2435 (0·7%)	1396 (0·9%)	1039 (0·6%)
American Indian or Alaska Native	724 (0·2%)	348 (0·2%)	375 (0·2%)
Native Hawaiian or other Pacific Islander	105 (<0·1%)	56 (<0·1%)	49 (<0·1%)
Multiple races	590 (0·2%)	301 (0·2%)	289 (0·2%)
Other race	4709 (1·4%)	2838 (1·7%)	1870 (1·1%)
Unknown race and ethnicity	75 334 (22·1%)	42 320 (25·7%)	32 999 (18·8%)

	Both mRNA vaccines (n=340 522)*	BNT162b2 vaccine (n=164 669)	mRNA-1273 vaccine (n=175 816)
(Continued from previous page)			
Signs or symptoms most frequently reported, non-serious‡			
Total	313 499	150 486	162 977
Headache	64 064 (20·4%)	30 907 (20·5%)	33 154 (20·3%)
Fatigue	52 048 (16·6%)	24 805 (16·5%)	27 241 (16·7%)
Pyrexia	51 023 (16·3%)	22 185 (14·7%)	28 837 (17·7%)
Chills	49 234 (15·7%)	21 638 (14·4%)	27 595 (16·9%)
Pain	47 745 (15·2%)	21 506 (14·3%)	26 238 (16·1%)
Nausea	37 333 (11·9%)	18 066 (12·0%)	19 267 (11·8%)
Dizziness	37 257 (11·9%)	20 307 (13·5%)	16 950 (10·4%)
Pain in extremity	31 753 (10·1%)	14 098 (9·4%)	17 653 (10·8%)
Injection-site pain	28 949 (9·2%)	10 462 (7·0%)	18 487 (11·3%)
Injection-site erythema	22 351 (7·1%)	2991 (2·0%)	19 360 (11·9%)
Signs or symptoms most frequently reported, serious‡			
Total	27 023	14 183	12 839
Dyspnoea	4175 (15·4%)	2210 (15·6%)	1965 (15·3%)
Death§	3802 (14·1%)	1753 (12·4%)	2039 (15·9%)
Pyrexia	2986 (11·0%)	1469 (10·4%)	1517 (11·8%)
Fatigue	2608 (9·7%)	1395 (9·8%)	1213 (9·4%)
Headache	2567 (9·5%)	1360 (9·6%)	1207 (9·4%)
Chest pain	2300 (8·5%)	1310 (9·2%)	990 (7·7%)
Nausea	2228 (8·2%)	1160 (8·2%)	1068 (8·3%)
Pain	2222 (8·2%)	1195 (8·4%)	1027 (8·0%)
Asthenia	2194 (8·1%)	1084 (7·6%)	1110 (8·6%)
Dizziness	2069 (7·7%)	1111 (7·8%)	958 (7·5%)

Data are n or n (%). Includes vaccines administered from Dec 14, 2020, to June 14, 2021. VAERS=Vaccine Adverse Event Reporting System. MedDRA=Medical Dictionary for Regulatory Activities. *Total includes reports without a vaccine manufacturer listed. †Race is not reported for individuals who identify as Hispanic or Latino, but it is reported for individuals with unknown ethnicity or non-Hispanic ethnicity. ‡Signs or symptoms refer to MedDRA preferred terms and are ordered by most frequently reported for both vaccines; MedDRA preferred terms are not mutually exclusive. §Not all reports of death were coded with the MedDRA preferred term of death.

Table 1: Characteristics of reports received and processed by VAERS for mRNA COVID-19 vaccines

	Both mRNA vaccines (n=4471*)		BNT162b2 vaccine (n=2086)		mRNA-1273 vaccine (n=2385)	
	n (%)	Reports per million doses administered†	n (%)	Reports per million doses administered†	n (%)	Reports per million doses administered†
Sex						
Female	1906 (42·6%)	12·2	918 (44·0%)	10·6	988 (41·4%)	14·2
Male	2485 (55·6%)	18·5	1116 (53·5%)	15·1	1369 (57·4%)	22·6
Unknown‡	80 (1·8%)	··	52 (2·5%)	··	28 (1·2%)	—
Age, years						
16–17	6 (0·1%)	1·1	6 (0·3%)	1·1	··	··
18–29	51 (1·1%)	1·3	27 (1·3%)	1·1	24 (1·0%)	1·6
30–39	94 (2·1%)	2·4	50 (2·4%)	2·2	44 (1·8%)	2·8
40–49	151 (3·4%)	3·8	74 (3·5%)	3·2	77 (3·2%)	4·6
50–59	328 (7·3%)	6·9	132 (6·3%)	5·0	196 (8·2%)	9·3
60–69	765 (17·1%)	14·4	354 (17·0%)	13·0	411 (17·2%)	16·0
70–79	1117 (25·0%)	28·5	496 (23·8%)	25·9	621 (26·0%)	31·0
80–89	1128 (25·2%)	75·4	529 (25·4%)	72·1	599 (25·1%)	78·6
≥90	637 (14·2%)	207·7	302 (14·5%)	188·1	335 (14·0%)	229·3
Unknown‡	194 (4·3%)	··	116 (5·6%)	··	78 (3·3%)	··

Includes reports made and vaccines administered from Dec 14, 2020, to June 14, 2021. VAERS=Vaccine Adverse Event Reporting System. *Of 4496 deaths, 25 were excluded as they could not be confirmed or were duplicate reports upon review. †Doses of vaccine administered in the study period were used for denominators in each age group; does not include doses administered in Texas because data for Texas were reported to the US Centers for Disease Control and Prevention in aggregate. ‡Reporting rates not shown for unknown categories because of unreliable dose denominators.

Table 3: Frequency and rates of death reported to VAERS by recipients of mRNA COVID-19 vaccines, by sex and age group

	Both mRNA vaccines		BNT162b2 vaccine		mRNA-1273 vaccine	
	Dose one (n=6 775 515)	Dose two (n=5 674 420)	Dose one (n=3 455 778)	Dose two (n=2 920 526)	Dose one (n=3 319 737)	Dose two (n=2 753 894)
Any injection-site reaction*	4 644 989 (68·6%)	4 068 447 (71·7%)	2 212 051 (64·0%)	1 908 124 (65·3%)	2 432 938 (73·3%)	2 160 323 (78·4%)
Injection-site pain	4 488 402 (66·2%)	3 890 848 (68·6%)	2 140 843 (61·9%)	1 835 398 (62·8%)	2 347 559 (70·7%)	2 055 450 (74·6%)
Swelling	703 790 (10·4%)	976 946 (17·2%)	246 230 (7·1%)	309 718 (10·6%)	457 560 (13·8%)	667 228 (24·2%)
Redness	353 788 (5·2%)	640 739 (11·3%)	116 108 (3·4%)	167 127 (5·7%)	237 680 (7·2%)	473 612 (17·2%)
Itching	376 076 (5·6%)	605 633 (10·7%)	145 596 (4·2%)	191 132 (6·5%)	230 480 (6·9%)	414 501 (15·1%)
Any systemic reaction*	3 573 429 (52·7%)	4 018 920 (70·8%)	1 771 509 (51·3%)	1 931 643 (66·1%)	1 801 920 (54·3%)	2 087 277 (75·8%)
Fatigue	2 295 205 (33·9%)	3 158 299 (55·7%)	1 127 904 (32·6%)	1 475 646 (50·5%)	1 167 301 (35·2%)	1 682 653 (61·1%)
Headache	1 831 471 (27·0%)	2 623 721 (46·2%)	893 992 (25·9%)	1 189 444 (40·7%)	937 479 (28·2%)	1 434 277 (52·1%)
Myalgia	1 423 336 (21·0%)	2 478 170 (43·7%)	653 821 (18·9%)	1 085 365 (37·2%)	769 515 (23·2%)	1 392 805 (50·6%)
Chills	631 546 (9·3%)	1 680 185 (29·6%)	263 617 (7·6%)	642 856 (22·0%)	367 929 (11·1%)	1 037 329 (37·7%)
Fever	642 092 (9·5%)	1 679 577 (29·6%)	274 650 (7·9%)	656 454 (22·5%)	367 442 (11·1%)	1 023 123 (37·2%)
Joint pain	642 006 (9·5%)	1 440 927 (25·4%)	285 812 (8·3%)	591 877 (20·3%)	356 194 (10·7%)	849 050 (30·8%)
Nausea	562 273 (8·3%)	901 103 (15·9%)	267 160 (7·7%)	384 525 (13·2%)	295 113 (8·9%)	516 578 (18·8%)
Diarrhoea	383 576 (5·7%)	419 044 (7·4%)	190 542 (5·5%)	198 618 (6·8%)	193 034 (5·8%)	220 426 (8·0%)
Abdominal pain	233 511 (3·4%)	359 107 (6·3%)	113 872 (3·3%)	158 251 (5·4%)	119 639 (3·6%)	200 856 (7·3%)
Rash	85 766 (1·3%)	99 878 (1·8%)	41 565 (1·2%)	42 662 (1·5%)	44 201 (1·3%)	57 216 (2·1%)
Vomiting	55 710 (0·8%)	91 727 (1·6%)	25 336 (0·7%)	36 761 (1·3%)	30 374 (0·9%)	54 966 (2·0%)
With reported health impacts*	808 963 (11·9%)	1 821 421 (32·1%)	361 834 (10·5%)	740 529 (25·4%)	447 129 (13·5%)	1 080 892 (39·2%)
Unable to do normal activity	658 330 (9·7%)	1 501 679 (26·5%)	290 207 (8·4%)	598 584 (20·5%)	368 123 (11·1%)	903 095 (32·8%)
Unable to work	305 709 (4·5%)	911 366 (16·1%)	135 063 (3·9%)	360 411 (12·3%)	170 646 (5·1%)	550 955 (20·0%)
Reported medical care	56 647 (0·8%)	53 077 (0·9%)	27 358 (0·8%)	25 568 (0·9%)	29 289 (0·9%)	27 509 (1·0%)
Telehealth consultation	19 562 (0·3%)	19 770 (0·3%)	9318 (0·3%)	9238 (0·3%)	10 244 (0·3%)	10 532 (0·4%)
Clinic attendance	18 671 (0·3%)	16 793 (0·3%)	9109 (0·3%)	8487 (0·3%)	9562 (0·3%)	8306 (0·3%)
Emergency room visit	9907 (0·1%)	8907 (0·2%)	5087 (0·1%)	4494 (0·2%)	4820 (0·1%)	4413 (0·2%)
Hospitalisation	1896 (<0·1%)	2053 (<0·1%)	915 (<0·1%)	1001 (<0·1%)	981 (<0·1%)	1052 (<0·1%)

Data are n (%). Includes health check-in surveys made and vaccines administered from Dec 14, 2020, to June 14, 2021. *Reports of local and systemic reactions and reported health impacts are not mutually exclusive.

Table 5: Local and systemic reactions and health impacts following mRNA COVID-19 vaccines reported during days 0–7 after vaccination to v-safe, by manufacturer and dose

21

	Both mRNA vaccines (n=298 792 852)		BNT162b2 vaccine (n=167 177 332)		mRNA-1273 vaccine (n=131 639 515)	
	n	Reports per million doses administered	n	Reports per million doses administered	n	Reports per million doses administered
Non-serious adverse event reports	313 499	1049·2	150 486	900·2	162 977	1238·1
Serious reports, including death	27 023	90·4	14 183	84·8	12 839	97·5
Serious reports, excluding death	22 527	75·4	12 078	72·2	10 448	79·4
Reports of adverse events of special interest*†						
COVID-19	9344	31·3	7184	43·0	2160	16·4
Coagulopathy‡	4320	14·5	2343	14·0	1977	15·0
Seizure	2733	9·1	1478	8·8	1255	9·5
Stroke§	1937	6·5	981	5·9	955	7·3
Bells' palsy	1918	6·4	1057	6·3	861	6·5
Anaphylaxis	1639	5·5	972	5·8	667	5·1
Myopericarditis	1307	4·4	813	4·9	494	3·8
Acute myocardial infarction	1118	3·7	610	3·6	508	3·9
Appendicitis	383	1·3	258	1·5	125	1·0
Guillain-Barré syndrome	293	1·0	154	0·9	139	1·1
Multisystem inflammatory syndrome in adults	119	0·4	60	0·4	59	0·4
Transverse myelitis	98	0·3	55	0·3	43	0·3
Narcolepsy	21	0·1	12	0·1	9	0·1

Includes vaccines administered from Dec 14, 2020, to June 14, 2021. VAERS=Vaccine Adverse Event Reporting System. *Represents reports, not confirmed by case definition. Events are not mutually exclusive. †Reported death is an adverse event of special interest but counts appear in tables 1 and 3. ‡Coagulopathy is an aggregate term capturing three specific adverse events: thrombocytopenia, deep venous thrombosis or pulmonary embolism, and disseminated intravascular coagulopathy. §No vaccine manufacturer was provided for one report of stroke.

Table 2: Frequency and rates of adverse events of special interest reported to VAERS by recipients of mRNA COVID-19 vaccines

	Both mRNA vaccines		BNT162b2 vaccine		mRNA-1273 vaccine	
	Dose one (n=6 775 515)	Dose two (n=5 674 420)	Dose one (n=3 455 778)	Dose two (n=2 920 526)	Dose one (n=3 319 737)	Dose two (n=2 753 894)
Any injection-site reaction*	4 644 989 (68·6%)	4 068 447 (71·7%)	2 212 051 (64·0%)	1 908 124 (65·3%)	2 432 938 (73·3%)	2 160 323 (78·4%)
Injection-site pain	4 488 402 (66·2%)	3 890 848 (68·6%)	2 140 843 (61·9%)	1 835 398 (62·8%)	2 347 559 (70·7%)	2 055 450 (74·6%)
Swelling	703 790 (10·4%)	976 946 (17·2%)	246 230 (7·1%)	309 718 (10·6%)	457 560 (13·8%)	667 228 (24·2%)
Redness	353 788 (5·2%)	640 739 (11·3%)	116 108 (3·4%)	167 127 (5·7%)	237 680 (7·2%)	473 612 (17·2%)
Itching	376 076 (5·6%)	605 633 (10·7%)	145 596 (4·2%)	191 132 (6·5%)	230 480 (6·9%)	414 501 (15·1%)
Any systemic reaction*	3 573 429 (52·7%)	4 018 920 (70·8%)	1 771 509 (51·3%)	1 931 643 (66·1%)	1 801 920 (54·3%)	2 087 277 (75·8%)
Fatigue	2 295 205 (33·9%)	3 158 299 (55·7%)	1 127 904 (32·6%)	1 475 646 (50·5%)	1 167 301 (35·2%)	1 682 653 (61·1%)
Headache	1 831 471 (27·0%)	2 623 721 (46·2%)	893 992 (25·9%)	1 189 444 (40·7%)	937 479 (28·2%)	1 434 277 (52·1%)
Myalgia	1 423 336 (21·0%)	2 478 170 (43·7%)	653 821 (18·9%)	1 085 365 (37·2%)	769 515 (23·2%)	1 392 805 (50·6%)
Chills	631 546 (9·3%)	1 680 185 (29·6%)	263 617 (7·6%)	642 856 (22·0%)	367 929 (11·1%)	1 037 329 (37·7%)
Fever	642 092 (9·5%)	1 679 577 (29·6%)	274 650 (7·9%)	656 454 (22·5%)	367 442 (11·1%)	1 023 123 (37·2%)
Joint pain	642 006 (9·5%)	1 440 927 (25·4%)	285 812 (8·3%)	591 877 (20·3%)	356 194 (10·7%)	849 050 (30·8%)
Nausea	562 273 (8·3%)	901 103 (15·9%)	267 160 (7·7%)	384 525 (13·2%)	295 113 (8·9%)	516 578 (18·8%)
Diarrhoea	383 576 (5·7%)	419 044 (7·4%)	190 542 (5·5%)	198 618 (6·8%)	193 034 (5·8%)	220 426 (8·0%)
Abdominal pain	233 511 (3·4%)	359 107 (6·3%)	113 872 (3·3%)	158 251 (5·4%)	119 639 (3·6%)	200 856 (7·3%)
Rash	85 766 (1·3%)	99 878 (1·8%)	41 565 (1·2%)	42 662 (1·5%)	44 201 (1·3%)	57 216 (2·1%)
Vomiting	55 710 (0·8%)	91 727 (1·6%)	25 336 (0·7%)	36 761 (1·3%)	30 374 (0·9%)	54 966 (2·0%)
With reported health impacts*	808 963 (11·9%)	1 821 421 (32·1%)	361 834 (10·5%)	740 529 (25·4%)	447 129 (13·5%)	1 080 892 (39·2%)
Unable to do normal activity	658 330 (9·7%)	1 501 679 (26·5%)	290 207 (8·4%)	598 584 (20·5%)	368 123 (11·1%)	903 095 (32·8%)
Unable to work	305 709 (4·5%)	911 366 (16·1%)	135 063 (3·9%)	360 411 (12·3%)	170 646 (5·1%)	550 955 (20·0%)
Reported medical care	56 647 (0·8%)	53 077 (0·9%)	27 358 (0·8%)	25 568 (0·9%)	29 289 (0·9%)	27 509 (1·0%)
Telehealth consultation	19 562 (0·3%)	19 770 (0·3%)	9318 (0·3%)	9238 (0·3%)	10 244 (0·3%)	10 532 (0·4%)
Clinic attendance	18 671 (0·3%)	16 793 (0·3%)	9109 (0·3%)	8487 (0·3%)	9562 (0·3%)	8306 (0·3%)
Emergency room visit	9907 (0·1%)	8907 (0·2%)	5087 (0·1%)	4494 (0·2%)	4820 (0·1%)	4413 (0·2%)
Hospitalisation	1896 (<0·1%)	2053 (<0·1%)	915 (<0·1%)	1001 (<0·1%)	981 (<0·1%)	1052 (<0·1%)

Data are n (%). Includes health check-in surveys made and vaccines administered from Dec 14, 2020, to June 14, 2021. *Reports of local and systemic reactions and reported health impacts are not mutually exclusive.

Table 5: Local and systemic reactions and health impacts following mRNA COVID-19 vaccines reported during days 0–7 after vaccination to v-safe, by manufacturer and dose

"From Dec 14, 2020, to June 14, 2021, 298 792 852 doses of mRNA COVID-19 vaccines were administered in the USA: 167 177 332 were BNT162b2 and 131 639 515 were mRNA-1273 (appendix p 2). A greater proportion of vaccines was administered to females (155 969 573 [53·2%]) than to males (134 373 958 [45·8%]). The median age at vaccination was 50 years (IQR 33–65) for BNT162b2 and 56 years (39–68) for mRNA-1273. 112 698 875 (38·4%) recipients were non-Hispanic White. Race and ethnicity was unknown for 102 227 532 (34·9%) of all vaccine recipients. During the study period, VAERS received and processed 340 522 reports: 164 669 following BNT162b2 and 175 816 following mRNA-1273 vaccination (table 1). Of these reports, 313 499 (92·1%) were classified as non-serious; 22 527 (6·6%) were serious, not resulting in death; and 4496 (1·3%) were deaths (table 1). 246 085 (72·3%) reports were among female participants and 154 171 (45·3%) reports were among those aged 18–49 years; median age was 50 years (IQR 36–64; table 1). 169 877 (49·9%) of those reporting race or ethnicity identified as non-Hispanic White, and for 75 334 (22·1%) race and ethnicity were unknown (table 1). The most common MedDRA preferred terms assigned to non-serious reports were headache (64 064 [20·4%] of 313 499), fatigue (52 048 [16·6%]), pyrexia (51 023 [16·3%]), chills (49 234 [15·7%]), and pain (47 745 [15·2%];

table 1). The most common MedDRA preferred terms assigned to serious reports were dyspnoea (4175 [15·4%] of 27023), death (3802 [14·1%]), pyrexia (2986 [11·0%]), fatigue (2608 [9·7%]), and headache (2567 [9·5%]; table 1)." (Source: Safety of mRNA vaccines administered during the initial 6 months of the US COVID-19 vaccination programme: an observational study of reports to the Vaccine Adverse Event Reporting System and v-safe (thelancet.com))

Table 2

Association between myocarditis and pericarditis and exposure to mRNA vaccines within 1 to 7 days and 8 to 21 days.

		Myocarditis				Pericarditis			
		Cases	Controls	OR (95% CI)[a]	aOR (95% CI)[b]	Cases	Controls	OR (95% CI)[a]	aOR (95% CI)[b]
Unexposed	Days[c]	1078	13342	Reference	Reference	1269	13398	Reference	Reference
BNT162b2									
Dose 1	1–7	51	370	1.7 (1.3–2.4)	1.8 (1.3–2.5)	43	398	1.1 (0.83–1.6)	1.3 (0.92–1.8)
	8–21	71	855	1.1 (0.86–1.4)	1.2 (0.93–1.6)	72	824	0.94 (0.73–1.2)	0.93 (0.72–1.2)
Dose 2	1–7	211	439	6.9 (5.7–8.4)	8.1 (6.7–9.9)	93	374	2.7 (2.2–3.5)	2.9 (2.3–3.8)
	8–21	72	816	1.2 (0.95–1.6)	1.3 (0.98–1.7)	80	765	1.2 (0.91–1.5)	1.3 (0.98–1.6)
mRNA-1273									
Dose 1	1–7	9	48	2.4 (1.2–5)	3 (1.4–6.2)	8	78	1.1 (0.52–2.2)	1.2 (0.56–2.4)
	8–21	10	109	1.2 (0.63–2.3)	1.1 (0.55–2.3)	9	146	0.65 (0.33–1.3)	0.73 (0.37–1.4)
Dose 2	1–7	106	51	27 (19–39)	30 (21–43)	26	54	5.3 (3.3–8.4)	5.5 (3.3–9)
	8–21	4	89	0.68 (0.25–1.9)	0.59 (0.19–1.9)	11	89	1.4 (0.72–2.5)	1.5 (0.76–2.9)
History of myocarditis or pericarditis[d]									
No		1486	16111	Reference	Reference	1440	16122	Reference	Reference
Yes		126	9	140 (71–280)	160 (83–330)	173	8	250 (120–520)	250 (120–540)
History of SARS-CoV-2 infection[e]									
No		1548	16013	Reference	Reference	1571	16020	Reference	Reference
Yes		64	107	6.3 (4.6–8.6)	9 (6.4–13)	42	110	3.9 (2.7–5.7)	4 (2.7–5.9)
Deprivation Index[f]									
Most deprived		986	9567	Reference	Reference	1049	10080	Reference	Reference
Least deprived		626	6553	0.9 (0.8–1)	0.88 (0.77–1)	564	6050	0.87 (0.77–0.98)	0.87 (0.76–0.99)

[a]Odds-ratio (95% confidence interval) were obtained from univariable conditional logistic regression, adjusting for matching variables (sex, age and department of residence).

[b]Adjusted odds-ratio (95% confidence interval) were obtained from multivariable conditional logistic regression, adjusting for all covariates and matching variables.

[c]Period of vaccine receipt relative to index date.

[d]Defined as an hospitalization with the respective condition within past 5 years.

[e]Either a positive RT-PCR or antigenic test for SARS-CoV-2, or hospitalization for COVID-19, within 30 days prior to index date.

[f]Least deprived refers to the grouping of 1st and 2nd quintiles, and most deprived to the grouping of 3d to 5th quintiles of the deprivation index.

Table 3

Description of hospitalized patients according to the exposure to mRNA vaccines.

	Myocarditis			Pericarditis		
	Unexposed	Vaccinated within 1 to 7 days	Vaccinated within 8 to 21 days	Unexposed	Vaccinated within 1 to 7 days	Vaccinated within 8 to 21 days
	(N = 1077)	(N = 378)	(N = 157)	(N = 1267)	(N = 172)	(N = 174)
Sex						
Male	829 (77.0)	324 (85.7)	128 (81.5)	778 (61.4)	101 (58.7)	110 (63.2)
Female	248 (23.0)	54 (14.3)	29 (18.5)	489 (38.6)	71 (41.3)	64 (36.8)
Age[a]						
Mean (sd)	28.5 (9.74)	25.6 (8.44)	28.6 (9.53)	33.8 (10.3)	29.9 (10.0)	33.9 (10.0)
Median (range)	26.0 (21.0-36.0)	23.0 (19.0-30.8)	26.0 (20.0-37.0)	35.0 (25.0-43.0)	29.0 (21.0-38.0)	34.0 (26.0-42.0)
Age distribution[a]						
12-17	114 (10.6)	40 (10.6)	12 (7.6)	80 (6.3)	12 (7.0)	9 (5.2)
18-24	356 (33.1)	171 (45.2)	59 (37.6)	228 (18.0)	56 (32.6)	28 (16.1)
25-29	168 (15.6)	60 (15.9)	22 (14.0)	152 (12.0)	22 (12.8)	23 (13.2)
30-39	248 (23.0)	74 (19.6)	39 (24.8)	361 (28.5)	47 (27.3)	57 (32.8)
40-50	191 (17.7)	33 (8.7)	25 (15.9)	446 (35.2)	35 (20.3)	57 (32.8)
Deprivation Index[b]						
Most deprived	654 (60.7)	237 (62.7)	95 (60.5)	820 (64.7)	115 (66.9)	114 (65.5)
Least deprived	423 (39.3)	141 (37.3)	62 (39.5)	447 (35.3)	57 (33.1)	60 (34.5)
History of myocarditis or pericarditis[c]	104 (9.7)	12 (3.2)	10 (6.4)	149 (11.8)	10 (5.8)	14 (8.0)
History of SARS-CoV-2 infection[d]	58 (5.4)	2 (0.5)	4 (2.5)	39 (3.1)	0 (0)	3 (1.7)
Length of hospital stay						
Mean (sd)	4.56 (5.97)	3.75 (2.60)	4.18 (2.70)	2.84 (4.46)	2.36 (2.49)	2.52 (2.84)
Median (range)	4.00 (2.00-5.00)	4.00 (2.00-5.00)	4.00 (3.00-5.00)	1.00 (0-4.00)	2.00 (1.00-4.00)	2.00 (1.00-3.00)
Death up to 30 days after discharge	4 (0.4)	0 (0)	0 (0)	4 (0.3)	0 (0)	1 (0.6)
among which deceased during hospital stay	3 (0.3)	0 (0)	0 (0)	1 (0.1)	0 (0)	1 (0.6)
Intensive care unit	66 (6.1)	9 (2.4)	6 (3.8)	32 (2.5)	0 (0)	2 (1.1)
Ventilation - oxygen therapy	46 (4.3)	12 (3.2)	5 (3.2)	30 (2.4)	1 (0.6)	3 (1.7)
Pericardial drainage	3 (0.3)	0 (0)	0 (0)	38 (3.0)	1 (0.6)	2 (1.1)

[a]At index date (date of hospital admission for myocarditis or pericarditis).

[b]Least deprived refers to the grouping of 1st and 2nd quintiles, and most deprived to the grouping of 3d to 5th quintiles of the deprivation index.

[c]Defined as an hospitalization with the respective condition within past 5 years.

[d]Either a positive RT-PCR or antigenic test for SARS-CoV-2, or hospitalization for COVID-19, within 30-days prior to index date.

Source: Age and sex-specific risks of myocarditis and pericarditis following Covid-19 messenger RNA vaccines - PMC (nih.gov) Table - PMC (nih.gov)

Source: CDC & FDA Identify Preliminary COVID-19 Vaccine Safety Signal for Persons Aged 65 Years and Older | CDC

Source: Myocarditis and Pericarditis After mRNA COVID-19 Vaccination | CDC

Straight From The CDC:

"CDC is providing timely updates on the following adverse events of interest:

- **Anaphylaxis after COVID-19 vaccination is rare** and has occurred at a rate of approximately 5 cases per one million vaccine doses administered. Anaphylaxis, a severe type of allergic reaction, can occur after any kind of vaccination. If it happens, healthcare providers can effectively and immediately treat the reaction. Learn more about COVID-19 vaccines and allergic reactions, including anaphylaxis.

CDC scientists have conducted detailed reviews of cases of anaphylaxis and made the information available to healthcare providers and the public:

  - Allergic Reactions Including Anaphylaxis After Receipt of the First Dose of Pfizer-BioNTech COVID-19 Vaccine

  - Reports of Anaphylaxis After Receipt of mRNA COVID-19 Vaccines in the US—December 14, 2020-January 18, 2021

  - Allergic Reactions Including Anaphylaxis After Receipt of the First Dose of Moderna COVID-19 Vaccine— United States, December 21, 2020-January 10, 2021

  - Allergic Reactions Including Anaphylaxis After Receipt of the First Dose of Pfizer-BioNTech COVID-19 Vaccine — United States, December 14-23, 2020

- **Thrombosis with thrombocytopenia syndrome (TTS) after J&J/Janssen COVID-19 vaccination is rare** and has occurred in approximately 4 cases per one million doses administered. TTS is a rare but serious adverse event that causes blood clots in large blood vessels and low platelets (blood cells that help form clots).

A review of reports indicates a causal relationship between the J&J/Janssen COVID-19 vaccine and TTS. CDC scientists have conducted detailed reviews of TTS cases and made the information available to healthcare providers and the public:

  - US Case Reports of Cerebral Venous Sinus Thrombosis With Thrombocytopenia After Ad26.COV2.S Vaccination, March 2 to April 21, 2021

  - Case Series of Thrombosis with Thrombocytopenia Syndrome following COVID-19 vaccination—United States, December 2020–August 2021

  - Updates on Thrombosis with Thrombocytopenia Syndrome (TTS) [1.3 MB, 39 Pages]

- **Guillain-Barré Syndrome (GBS) in people who have received the J&J/Janssen COVID-19 vaccine is rare.** GBS is a rare disorder where the body's immune system damages nerve cells, causing muscle weakness and sometimes paralysis. GBS has largely been reported in men ages 50 years and older.

Based on a recent analysis of data from the Vaccine Safety Datalink, the rate of GBS within the first 21 days following J&J/Janssen COVID-19 vaccination was found to be 21 times higher than after Pfizer-BioNTech or Moderna (mRNA COVID-19 vaccines). After the first 42 days, the rate of GBS was 11 times higher following J&J/Janssen COVID-19 vaccination.

The analysis found no increased risk of GBS after Pfizer-BioNTech or Moderna (mRNA COVID-19 vaccines). CDC and FDA will continue to monitor for and evaluate reports of GBS occurring after COVID-19 vaccination and will share more information as it becomes available.

• **Myocarditis and pericarditis after COVID-19 vaccination are rare.** Myocarditis is inflammation of the heart muscle, and pericarditis is inflammation of the outer lining of the heart. Most patients with myocarditis or pericarditis after COVID-19 vaccination responded well to medicine and rest and felt better quickly. Most cases have been reported after receiving Pfizer-BioNTech or Moderna (mRNA COVID-19 vaccines), particularly in male adolescents and young adults.

A review of vaccine safety data in VAERS from December 2020–August 2021 found a small but increased risk of myocarditis after mRNA COVID-19 vaccines. Over 350 million mRNA vaccines were given during the study period and CDC scientists found that rates of myocarditis were highest following the second dose of an mRNA vaccine among males in the following age groups:

- 12–15 years (70.7 cases per one million doses of Pfizer-BioNTech)

- 16–17 years (105.9 cases per one million doses of Pfizer-BioNTech)

- 18–24 years (52.4 cases and 56.3 cases per million doses of Pfizer-BioNTech and Moderna, respectively)

  Multiple studies and reviews of data from vaccine safety monitoring systems continue to show that vaccines are safe. As a result, the agency will refocus enhanced surveillance and safety monitoring efforts toward children and adolescents.

  As of January 26, 2023, there have been 1,060 preliminary reports in VAERS among people younger than age 18 years under review for potential cases of myocarditis and pericarditis. Of these, 247 remain under review. Through confirmation of symptoms and diagnostics by provider interview or review of medical records, 710 reports have been verified to meet CDC's working case definition for myocarditis. See below for counts of verified reports of myocarditis by age group.

- 5-11 years: 23 verified reports of myocarditis after 23,178,311 doses administered

- 12-15 years: 371 verified reports of myocarditis after 25,791,756 doses administered

- 16-17 years: 316 verified reports of myocarditis after 14,117,149 doses administered

  As the COVID-19 vaccines are authorized for younger children, CDC and FDA will continue to monitor for and evaluate reports of myocarditis and pericarditis after COVID-19 vaccination and will share more information as it becomes available. Learn more about myocarditis and pericarditis, including clinical considerations, after mRNA COVID-19 vaccination.

• **Reports of death after COVID-19 vaccination** are rare. FDA requires healthcare providers to report any death after COVID-19 vaccination to VAERS, even if it's unclear whether the vaccine was the cause. **Reports of adverse events to VAERS following vaccination, including deaths, do not necessarily mean that a vaccine caused a health problem.** More than 668 million doses of COVID-19 vaccines were administered in the United States from December 14, 2020, through January 26, 2023. During this time, VAERS received 18,977 preliminary reports of death (0.0028%) among people who received a COVID-19 vaccine. CDC and FDA clinicians review reports of death to VAERS including death certificates, autopsy, and medical records. Continued monitoring has identified nine deaths causally associated with J&J/Janssen COVID-19 vaccination. CDC and FDA continue to review reports of death following COVID-19 vaccination and update information as it becomes available."

Source: Selected Adverse Events Reported after COVID-19 Vaccination | CDC

Blog Post - Click Here:
Over 1,000 Scientific Studies That Prove The COVID-19 Vaccines Are Dangerous (zinglepathy.com)

UNDISCLOSED COVID-19 VACCINE INGREDIENTS LIST

Undisclosed Covid-19 Vaccine Ingredients List:

Non-disclosed Ingredients	Pfizer/Biontech	Moderna	Janssen (JNJ)	AstraZeneca	Toxicological Symptoms:	Detox With:
Aluminum [nanoparticles]	YES	YES			Neurotoxin – can sneak past the blood-brain barrier with ease: Alzheimer's disease, amyotrophic lateral sclerosis, anemia and other blood disorders, colic, fatigue, dementia dialectica, kidney and liver dysfunctions, neuromuscular disorders, osteomalacia, Parkinson's disease	BioSil, Enterosgel, Zeolite
Bismuth [nanoparticles]	YES				Gingivitis, Loss of weight, Loss of appetite, Albuminuria (the presence of albumin in the urine, typically as a symptom of kidney disease.), Diarrhea, Skin reactions, Skin allergies to cosmetics & personal use products, Headaches, Fever, Depression, Kidney disease, Liver damage, Anemia, Ulcerative stomatitis, Dermatitis	
Cadmium [nanoparticles]		YES			This highly toxic nano particulate composition are quantum dots of cadmium selenide which are cytotoxic and genotoxic. Hypertension, arthritis, diabetes, anemia, arteriosclerosis, impaired bone healing, cancer, cardiovascular disease, cirrhosis, reduced fertility, hyperlipidemia, hypoglycemia, headaches, osteoporosis, kidney disease, schizophrenia, and strokes.	Zeolite
Calcium		YES				
Carbon [nanoparticles]	YES	YES			Highly magnetic and can trigger pathological blood coagulation and "The Corona Effect" or "The Spike Protein Effect" creation from the degeneration of the cell membrane due to interactions with other dipoles. 'The CORONA EFFECT' on the red blood cells with showing 'The SPIKED PROTEIN EFFECT' both caused by decompensated acidosis of the interstitial and then vascular fluids from an acidic lifestyle and specifically, exposure to toxic pulsating electro-magnetic fields at 2.4gHz or higher, chemical poisoning from the food and water ingested, toxic acidic air pollution, chem-trails and to top-it-all-off a nano particulate chemical laden CoV – 19 inoculation.	Star Anise/Fennel, C60, Pine Needle Tea, Schizandra Berry, St. John's Wort, Gingko Biloba Leaf, Quercetin/HCQ, Ivermectin, Dandelion Leaf, Chlorine Dioxide (CDS)
Chloride	YES					
Chlorine (From Saline Solution)	YES	YES	YES	YES		
Chromium	YES		YES	YES	Weight loss, anemia, thrombocytopenia, liver dysfunction, renal failure, rhabdomyolysis, dermatitis, and hypoglycemia	Zeolite
Copper [nanoparticles]	YES	YES		YES	Acne, adrenal hyperactivity and/or insufficiency, agoraphobia, allergies, hair loss, anemia, anxiety, arthritis, autism, cancer, chronic candida albicans infection, depression, elevated cholesterol, cystic fibrosis, depression, diabetes, dyslexia, elevated estrogen, failure to thrive, fatigue, fears, fractures of the bones, headaches, heart attacks, hyperactivity, hypertension, hypothyroidism, infections, inflammation, insomnia, iron storage diseases, kidney and liver dysfunctions, decreased libido, multiple sclerosis, nervousness, osteoporosis, panic attacks, premenstrual syndrome, schizophrenia, strokes, tooth decay and vitamin C and other vitamin deficiencies.	
Ethylene Alcohol	YES	YES		YES	Carcinogenic and genotoxic.	
Graphene Oxide [GO]	YES	YES	YES	YES	Creates thromboses, causes blood clots, trigger cytokine storm, pneumonia, inflammation of the mucous membranes, passes through the blood-brain barrier.	Chlorine dioxide – neutralizes spikes, NAC/Glutathione – neutralizes GO. Raw Garlic Cloves detoxes GO
Iron [nanoparticles]	YES	YES	YES	YES		

Non-disclosed Ingredients	Pfizer/Biontech	Moderna	Janssen (JNJ)	AstraZeneca	Toxicological Symptoms:	Detox With:
Lead		YES			Abdominal pain, adrenal insufficiency, anemia, arthritis, arteriosclerosis, attention deficit, back problems, blindness, cancer, constipation, convulsions, deafness, depression, diabetes, dyslexia, epilepsy, fatigue, gout, impaired glycogen storage, hallucinations, hyperactivity, impotency, infertility, inflammation, kidney dysfunction, learning disabilities, diminished libido, migraine headaches, multiple sclerosis, psychosis, thyroid imbalances, and tooth decay.	Zeolite, Chlorella, Ecklonia Cava, Humic Fulvic Acid, Modified Citrus Pectin, Purified Silica
Magnesium		YES				Zeolite
Manganese			YES		Psychosis, impaired speech tremors, loss of coordination, muscular weakness	Zeolite
Nickel			YES	YES	Cancer (oral and intestinal), depression, heart attacks, hemorrhages, kidney dysfunction, low blood pressure, malaise, muscle tremors and paralysis, nausea, skin problems, tetany, and vomiting.	Zeolite
Nitrogen [nanoparticles]	YES	YES				
Oxygen [nanoparticles]	YES	YES				
Oxygen Chromium	YES					
Phosphorus [nanoparticles]	YES	YES				
Poly-Ethylene Glycol (PEG)	YES	YES		YES	Carcinogenic and genotoxic.	
Potassium		YES				
Selenium [nanoparticles]		YES			This highly toxic nano particulate composition are quantum dots of cadmium selenide which are cytotoxic and genotoxic.	
Silicon [nanoparticles]	YES	YES	YES	YES		
Sodium [From Saline Solution]	YES	YES	YES	YES		
Sulphur	YES			YES		Zeolite
Tin				YES		Zeolite, Iron, Calcium, Vitamin B2, Vitamin E, Zinc
Titanium	YES	YES			Lung diseases, Skin diseases (Eczema), Sinus congestion, Cancer, Vision problems, Sexual weakness (pre-mature ejaculation), Bright's disease (a disease involving chronic inflammation of the kidneys), Lupus (any of various diseases or conditions marked by inflammation of the skin).	
Trypanosoma Cruzi (parasite)	YES				Trypanosoma cruzi parasite of which several variants are lethal and is one of many causes of acquired immune deficiency syndrome or AIDS. [Atlas of Human Parasitology, 4th Edition, Lawrence Ash and Thomas Orithel, pages 174 to 178]	Zeolite, Enterosgel, Activated Charcoal
Vanadium	YES				Toxic amounts of vanadium can range from loss of appetite and common digestive problems (e.g., nausea, vomiting, stomach pain, gas, diarrhea, and loose stool) to damage of the liver and nervous system, kidney failure and lack of growth. Other symptoms of vanadium toxicity include irritation of mucous membranes and the upper respiratory tract, inflammation of stomach and intestines, skin rash, nose bleeding and internal bleeding, dizziness and headaches, cardiovascular problems, and behavioral changes. High doses of vanadium may cause anemia, low white blood cell counts, sudden drop in blood sugar levels (hypoglycemia), high cholesterol, fertility problems and birth defects.	Zeolite

[Source: https://www.planet-today.com/2021/09/american-scientists-confirm-toxic.html#gsc.tab=0]

HISTORICALLY UTILIZED VACCINE INGREDIENTS - USED IN THE PAST &/OR CURRENTLY

Historically Utilized Vaccine Ingredients - Used In The Past &/or Currently:

Do you know what's in a vaccine?

- **ALUMINUM:** Implicated as a cause of brain damage. Suspected factor in ALZHEIMER's DISEASE, dementia, seizures, and comas.

Material Safety Data Sheet
Aluminum (Metallic, Powder)

ACC# 01000

Section 1 - Chemical Product and Company Identification

MSDS Name: Aluminum (Metallic, Powder)
Catalog Numbers: A559-500
Synonyms: None.
Company Identification:
    Fisher Scientific
    1 Reagent Lane
    Fair Lawn, NJ 07410
For information, call: 201-796-7100
Emergency Number: 201-796-7100
For CHEMTREC assistance, call: 800-424-9300
For International CHEMTREC assistance, call: 703-527-3887

Section 2 - Composition, Information on Ingredients

CAS#	Chemical Name	Percent	EINECS/ELINCS
7429-90-5	Aluminum	100	231-072-3

Section 3 - Hazards Identification

EMERGENCY OVERVIEW

Appearance: silver-gray powder.
Danger! Dust may form flammable or explosive mixture with air, especially when damp. Reacts violently and/or explosively with water, steam or moisture. May ignite or explode on contact with moist air. May cause eye and skin irritation. May cause respiratory tract irritation. Air sensitive.
Target Organs: Lungs, eyes, skin.

Potential Health Effects
Eye: May cause eye irritation.
Skin: May cause skin irritation. Low hazard for usual industrial handling. No sensitizing effects known.
Ingestion: May cause gastrointestinal irritation with nausea, vomiting and diarrhea.
Inhalation: May cause respiratory tract irritation. May cause respiratory difficulty and coughing.
Chronic: Aluminum may be implicated in Alzheimer's disease. Inhalation of aluminum containing dusts may cause pulmonary disease.

Aluminum	Adjuvant	Adacel	Tdap	0.33 mg
Aluminum	Adjuvant	Bexsero	Meningococcal Group B	0.519 mg
Aluminum	Adjuvant	BioThrax	Anthrax	1.2 mg/mL
Aluminum	Adjuvant	Boostrix	Tdap	≤0.39 mg
Aluminum	Adjuvant	Daptacel	DTaP	0.33 mg
Aluminum	Adjuvant	DT	DT	1.5 mg aluminum phosphate
Aluminum	Adjuvant	Engerix-B	HepB	0.5 mg/mL
Aluminum	Adjuvant	Gardasil	HPV	225 mcg
Aluminum	Adjuvant	Gardasil 9	HPV	500 mcg
Aluminum	Adjuvant	Havrix	HepA	0.5 mg/mL
Aluminum	Adjuvant	Infanrix	DTaP	≤0.625 mg
Aluminum	Adjuvant	Ixiaro	Japanese Encephalitis	250 mcg aluminum hydroxide
Aluminum	Adjuvant	Kinrix	DTaP+IPV	≤0.6 mg
Aluminum	Adjuvant	Pediarix	DTaP+HepB+IPV	≤0.85 mg
Aluminum	Adjuvant	PedvaxHIB	Hib+HepB	225 mcg
Aluminum	Adjuvant	Pentacel	DTaP+IPV+Hib	0.33 mg
Aluminum	Adjuvant	Prevnar 13	Pneumococcal 13-valent	125 mcg
Aluminum	Adjuvant	Quadracel	DTaP+IPV	0.33 mg
Aluminum	Adjuvant	Recombivax HB	HepB	0.5 mg/mL
Aluminum	Adjuvant	Td (generic)	Td	≤0.53 mg
Aluminum	Adjuvant	Tenivac	Td	0.33 mg
Aluminum	Adjuvant	Trumenba	Meningococcal Group B	0.25 mg
Aluminum	Adjuvant	Twinrix	HepA+HepB	0.45 mg
Aluminum	Adjuvant	Vaqta	HepA	0.45 mg

- **AMMONIUM SULFATE:** Suspected as a poison that can cause major damage to gastrointestinal, liver, nerve, and respiratory system.

- **BETA-PROPIOLACTONE:** Known to cause CANCER. Suspected as a poison that can cause major damage to gastrointestinal, liver, nerve, respiratory, skin, and other organs.

- **GELATIN:** Produced from selected pieces of calf and cattle skins, de-mineralized cattle bones, and pork skin. ALLERGIC reactions have been reported.

- **GENTAMICIN SULFATE & POLYMYXIN B [ANTIBIOTICS]:** ALLERGIC reactions can range from mild to life-threatening.

- **GENETICALLY MODIFIED YEAST, ANIMAL, BACTERIAL, & VIRAL DNA:** Can be incorporated into the recipient's DNA and cause unknown GENETIC MUTATIONS.

- **GLUTARALDEHYDE:** Poisonous if ingested. Causes BIRTH DEFECTS in experimental animals.
- **FORMALDEHYDE [FORMALIN]:** Major constituent of embalming fluid. Poisonous if ingested. Probable carcinogen. Suspected as a poison that can cause major damage to gastrointestinal, liver, respiratory, immune, nerve, and reproductive system.

FORMALDEHYDE, 37% SOLUTION
FORMALIN

POISON!   DANGER!

CAUSES BURNS. HARMFUL IF SWALLOWED, INHALED, OR ABSORBED THROUGH SKIN. MAY CAUSE ALLERGIC SKIN REACTION. COMBUSTIBLE.

Potential cancer hazard. Exercise due care. Keep away from heat, sparks, and flame. Do not get in eyes, on skin, or on clothing. Avoid breathing vapor. Keep in tightly closed container. Use with adequate ventilation. Wash thoroughly after handling.

PRECAUTIONARY STATEMENTS: Vapors may be irritating to skin, eyes, nose, and throat. Inhalation may cause severe irritation of the respiratory system. Contact with skin or eyes may cause severe irritation or burns. Ingestion may cause severe burning to mouth and stomach.

Level of formaldehyde   µg=mcg

Low – below 50 µg/m3 (40ppb) No adverse effects should be noticed.

Moderate – above 50 µg/m3 (40ppb) Long-term exposure may result in respiratory symptoms such as coughing and wheezing, and allergic sensitivity, especially in children.

High – above 123 µg/m3 (100 ppb) the risk of irritation or burning sensation in eyes, nose and throat from short-term exposure grows with increasing concentration. There is also an increased likelihood of respiratory symptoms from long-term exposure.

Formaldehyde	Inactivating Agent	ActHIB	Hib	<0.5 mcg	
Formaldehyde	Inactivating Agent	Adacel	Tdap	≤5 mcg	100mg=100,000µg
Formaldehyde	Preservative	BioThrax	Anthrax	100 mg/mL	
Formaldehyde	Inactivating Agent	Boostrix	Tdap	≤100 mcg (residual)	
Formaldehyde	Inactivating Agent	Daptacel	DTaP	≤5 mcg (residual)	
Formaldehyde	Inactivating Agent	DT	DT	<100 mcg	
Formaldehyde	Inactivating Agent	Fluad	Influenza	≤10 mcg	
Formaldehyde	Inactivating Agent	Fluarix Quad	Influenza	≤5 mcg	
Formaldehyde	Inactivating Agent	Flulaval Quad	Influenza	≤25 mcg	
Formaldehyde	Inactivating Agent	FluZone High Dose	Influenza	≤100 mcg	mcg= µg
Formaldehyde	Inactivating Agent	FluZone Intradermal	Influenza	≤20 mcg	
Formaldehyde	Inactivating Agent	FluZone Quad	Influenza	≤100 mcg	
Formaldehyde	Inactivating Agent	Havrix	HepA	≤0.1 mg formalin	
Formaldehyde	Inactivating Agent	Hiberix	Hib	<0.5 mcg (residual)	
Formaldehyde	Inactivating Agent	Infanrix	DTaP	≤100 mcg (residual)	
Formaldehyde	Inactivating Agent	IPOL	Polio	≤0.02%	
Formaldehyde	Inactivating Agent	Ixiaro	Japanese Encephalitis	≤200 pmm	
Formaldehyde	Inactivating Agent	JE-Vax	Japanese Encephalitis	<100 mcg	
Formaldehyde	Inactivating Agent	Kinrix	DTaP+IPV	≤100 mcg (residual)	
Formaldehyde	Inactivating Agent	Menactra	Meningococcal	<2.66 mcg	
Formaldehyde	Inactivating Agent	MenQuadfi	Meningococcal	<3 mcg/mL	
Formaldehyde	Inactivating Agent	Menveo	Meningococcal	≤0.30 mcg	
Formaldehyde	Inactivating Agent	Pediarix	DTaP+HepB+IPV	≤100 mcg (residual)	
Formaldehyde	Inactivating Agent	Pentacel	DTaP+IPV+Hib	≤2 mcg (residual)	
Formaldehyde	Inactivating Agent	Quadracel	DTaP+IPV	≤5 mcg	
Formaldehyde	Inactivating Agent	Recombivax HB	HepB	<15 mcg/mL (residual)	
Formaldehyde	Inactivating Agent	TDVAX	Td	100 mcg	
Formaldehyde	Inactivating Agent	Tenivac	Td	≤5 mcg (residual)	
Formaldehyde	Inactivating Agent	Twinrix	HepA+HepB	≤0.1 mg formalin	
Formaldehyde	Inactivating Agent	Typhim Vi	Typhoid	≤100 mcg (residual)	
Formaldehyde	Inactivating Agent	Vaqta	HepA	<0.8 mcg	

- **HUMAN & ANIMAL CELLS:** Human cells from aborted FETAL TISSUE and human albumin, pig blood, horse blood, rabbit brain, guinea pig, dog kidney, cow heart, monkey kidney, chicken embryo, chicken egg, duck egg, calf serum, sheep blood, and others. Aborted human diploid cell cultures (WI-38 & MRC-5).

- **LATEX RUBBER:** Can cause life-threatening allergic reactions.

- **MERCURY [THIMEROSAL]:** One of the most poisonous substances known. Has an affinity for the brain, gut, liver, bone marrow, and kidneys. Minute amounts can cause nerve damage. There is strong correlation between mercury toxicity and AUTISM.

- **MICRO-ORGANISMS:** Dead and alive virus and bacteria or their toxins. The polio vaccine was contaminated with a monkey virus (Simian Virus 40 – "SV40"), now turning up in human bone, lung-lining (mesothelioma), brain tumors, and lymphomas.

- **MONOSODIUM GLUTAMATE [MSG, GLUTAMATE, GLUTAMATE ACID]:** A NEUROTOXIN that's being studied for mutagenic, teratogenic (developmental and monstrosities) and reproductive effects. Allergic reactions can range from mild to severe.

- **NEOMYCIN SULFATE [ANTIBIOTIC]:** Interferes with vitamin B6 absorption. An error in the uptake of B6 can cause a rare form of epilepsy and mental retardation. Allergic reactions can range from mild to life threatening.

- **PHENOL/PHENOXYETHANOL [2-PE]:** Used as anti-freeze. TOXIC to all cells and capable of disabling the immune system's primary response mechanism.

- **POLYSORBATE 80:** Known to cause CANCER in animals.

- **TRI(N)BUTYLPHOSPHATE:** Suspected to be a poison to the kidney and nerves.

Don't believe me? Check out the CDC's Vaccine Excipient list below:

Vaccine Excipient Table

Vaccine (Trade Name)	Package Insert Date	Contains[a]
Adenovirus	10/2019	monosodium glutamate, sucrose, D-mannose, D-fructose, dextrose, human serum albumin, potassium phosphate, plasdone C, anhydrous lactose, microcrystalline cellulose, polacrilin potassium, magnesium stearate, cellulose acetate phthalate, alcohol, acetone, castor oil, FD&C Yellow #6 aluminum lake dye
Anthrax (Biothrax)	11/2015	aluminum hydroxide, sodium chloride, benzethonium chloride, formaldehyde
BCG (Tice)	02/2009	glycerin, asparagine, citric acid, potassium phosphate, magnesium sulfate, iron ammonium citrate, lactose
Cholera (Vaxchora)	06/2016	ascorbic acid, hydrolyzed casein, sodium chloride, sucrose, dried lactose, sodium bicarbonate, sodium carbonate
Dengue (Dengvaxia)	06/2019	sodium chloride, essential amino acids (including L-phenylalanine), non-essential amino acids, L-arginine hydrochloride, sucrose, D-trehalose dihydrate, D-sorbitol, trometamol, urea
DT (Sanofi)	06/2018	aluminum phosphate, isotonic sodium chloride, formaldehyde
DTaP (Daptacel)	01/2021[b]	aluminum phosphate, formaldehyde, glutaraldehyde, 2-phenoxyethanol
DTaP (Infanrix)	01/2021[b]	formaldehyde, aluminum hydroxide, sodium chloride, polysorbate 80 (Tween 80)
DTaP-IPV (Kinrix)	01/2021[b]	formaldehyde, aluminum hydroxide, sodium chloride, polysorbate 80 (Tween 80), neomycin sulfate, polymyxin B
DTaP-IPV (Quadracel)	02/2021	formaldehyde, aluminum phosphate, 2-phenoxyethanol, polysorbate 80, glutaraldehyde, neomycin, polymyxin B sulfate, bovine serum albumin
DTaP-HepB-IPV (Pediarix)	01/2021[b]	formaldehyde, aluminum hydroxide, aluminum phosphate, sodium chloride, polysorbate 80 (Tween 80), neomycin sulfate, polymyxin B, yeast protein
DTaP-IPV/Hib (Pentacel)	12/2019	aluminum phosphate, polysorbate 80, sucrose, formaldehyde, glutaraldehyde, bovine serum albumin, 2-phenoxyethanol, neomycin, polymyxin B sulfate
DTaP-IPV-Hib-HepB (Vaxelis)	10/2020	polysorbate 80, formaldehyde, glutaraldehyde, bovine serum albumin, neomycin, streptomycin sulfate, polymyxin B sulfate, ammonium thiocyanate, yeast protein, aluminum
Ebola Zaire (ERVEBO)	01/2021[b]	Tromethamine, rice-derived recombinant human serum albumin, host cell DNA, benzonase, rice protein
Hib (ActHIB)	05/2019	sodium chloride, formaldehyde, sucrose
Hib (Hiberix)	04/2018	formaldehyde, sodium chloride, lactose

Hib (PedvaxHIB)	01/2021[b]	amorphous aluminum hydroxyphosphate sulfate, sodium chloride
Hep A (Havrix)	01/2021[b]	MRC-5 cellular proteins, formalin, aluminum hydroxide, amino acid supplement, phosphate-buffered saline solution, polysorbate 20, neomycin sulfate, aminoglycoside antibiotic
Hep A (Vaqta)	01/2021[b]	amorphous aluminum hydroxyphosphate sulfate, non-viral protein, DNA, bovine albumin, formaldehyde, neomycin, sodium borate, sodium chloride, other process chemical residuals
Hep B (Engerix-B)	01/2021[b]	aluminum hydroxide, yeast protein, sodium chloride, disodium phosphate dihydrate, sodium dihydrogen phosphate dihydrate
Hep B (Recombivax)	12/2018	formaldehyde, potassium aluminum sulfate, amorphous aluminum hydroxyphosphate sulfate, yeast protein
Hep B (Heplisav-B)	05/2020	yeast protein, yeast DNA, deoxycholate, phosphorothioate linked oligodeoxynucleotide, sodium phosphate, dibasic dodecahydrate, sodium chloride, monobasic dehydrate, polysorbate 80
Hep A/Hep B (Twinrix)	01/2021[b]	MRC-5 cellular proteins, formalin, aluminum phosphate, aluminum hydroxide, amino acids, sodium chloride, phosphate buffer, polysorbate 20, neomycin sulfate, yeast protein
HPV (Gardasil 9)	08/2020	amorphous aluminum hydroxyphosphate sulfate, sodium chloride, L-histidine, polysorbate 80, sodium borate, yeast protein

Vaccine (Trade Name)	Package Insert Date	Contains[a]
Influenza (Afluria) Quadrivalent[c]	03/2021	sodium chloride, monobasic sodium phosphate, dibasic sodium phosphate, monobasic potassium phosphate, potassium chloride, calcium chloride, sodium taurodeoxycholate, ovalbumin, sucrose, neomycin sulfate, polymyxin B, beta-propiolactone, hydrocortisone, thimerosal (multi-dose vials)
Influenza (Fluad) Quadrivalent[c]	03/2021	squalene, polysorbate 80, sorbitan trioleate, sodium citrate dihydrate, citric acid monohydrate, neomycin, kanamycin, hydrocortisone, egg protein, formaldehyde
Influenza (Fluarix) Quadrivalent[c]	2021	octoxynol-10 (TRITON X-100), α-tocopheryl hydrogen succinate, polysorbate 80 (Tween 80), hydrocortisone, gentamicin sulfate, ovalbumin, formaldehyde, sodium deoxycholate, sodium phosphate-buffered isotonic sodium chloride
Influenza (Flublok) Quadrivalent[c]	03/2021	sodium chloride, monobasic sodium phosphate, dibasic sodium phosphate, polysorbate 20 (Tween 20), baculovirus and *Spodoptera frugiperda* cell proteins, baculovirus and cellular DNA, Triton X-100
Influenza (Flucelvax) Quadrivalent[c]	10/2021[b]	Madin Darby Canine Kidney (MDCK) cell protein, phosphate buffered saline, protein other than HA, MDCK cell DNA, polysorbate 80, cetyltrimethlyammonium bromide, and β-propiolactone, thimerosal (multi-dose vials)
Influenza (Flulaval) Quadrivalent[c]	2021	ovalbumin, formaldehyde, sodium deoxycholate, α-tocopheryl hydrogen succinate, polysorbate 80, phosphate-buffered saline solution
Influenza (Fluzone) Quadrivalent[c]	2021	formaldehyde, egg protein, octylphenol ethoxylate (Triton X-100), sodium phosphate-buffered isotonic sodium chloride solution, thimerosal (multi-dose vials)
Influenza (Fluzone) High Dose[c]	07/2021	egg protein, octylphenol ethoxylate (Triton X-100), sodium phosphate-buffered isotonic sodium chloride solution, formaldehyde
Influenza (FluMist) Quadrivalent[c]	08/2021	monosodium glutamate, hydrolyzed porcine gelatin, arginine, sucrose, dibasic potassium phosphate, monobasic potassium phosphate, ovalbumin, gentamicin sulfate, ethylenediaminetetraacetic acid (EDTA)
IPV (Ipol)	01/2021[b]	calf bovine serum albumin, 2-phenoxyethanol, formaldehyde, neomycin, streptomycin, polymyxin B, M-199 medium

Vaccine (Trade Name)	Package Insert Date	Contains[a]
Japanese Encephalitis (Ixiaro)	09/2018	aluminum hydroxide, protamine sulfate, formaldehyde, bovine serum albumin, host cell DNA, sodium metabisulphite, host cell protein
MenACWY (Menactra)	04/2018	sodium phosphate buffered isotonic sodium chloride solution, formaldehyde, diphtheria toxoid protein carrier
MenACWY (MenQuadfi)	01/2021[b]	sodium chloride, sodium acetate, formaldehyde
MenACWY (Menveo)	07/2020	formaldehyde, CRM$_{197}$ protein
MenB (Bexsero)	01/2021[b]	aluminum hydroxide, sodium chloride, histidine, sucrose, kanamycin
MenB (Trumenba)	2018	polysorbate 80, aluminum phosphate, histidine buffered saline
MMR (MMR-II)	12/2020	sorbitol, sucrose, hydrolyzed gelatin, recombinant human albumin, neomycin, fetal bovine serum, WI-38 human diploid lung fibroblasts
MMRV (ProQuad) (Frozen: Recombinant Albumin)	01/2021[b]	MRC-5 cells including DNA and protein, sucrose, hydrolyzed gelatin, sodium chloride, sorbitol, monosodium L-glutamate, sodium phosphate dibasic, recombinant human albumin, sodium bicarbonate, potassium phosphate monobasic, potassium chloride, potassium phosphate dibasic, neomycin, bovine calf serum, other buffer and media ingredients
PCV13 (Prevnar 13)	08/2017	CRM$_{197}$ carrier protein, polysorbate 80, succinate buffer, aluminum phosphate
PPSV-23 (Pneumovax)	09/2020	isotonic saline solution, phenol
Rabies (Imovax)	10/2019	human albumin, neomycin sulfate, phenol red, beta-propiolactone
Rabies (RabAvert)	2018	chicken protein, polygeline (processed bovine gelatin), human serum albumin, potassium glutamate, sodium EDTA, ovalbumin, neomycin, chlortetracycline, amphotericin B
Rotavirus (RotaTeq)	01/2021[b]	sucrose, sodium citrate, sodium phosphate monobasic monohydrate, sodium hydroxide, polysorbate 80, cell culture media, fetal bovine serum

Vaccine (Trade Name)	Package Insert Date	Contains[a]
Rotavirus (Rotarix)	01/2021[b]	dextran, Dulbecco's Modified Eagle Medium (sodium chloride, potassium chloride, magnesium sulfate, ferric (III) nitrate, sodium phosphate, sodium pyruvate, D-glucose, concentrated vitamin solution, L-cystine, L-tyrosine, amino acids, L-glutamine, calcium chloride, sodium hydrogenocarbonate, and phenol red), sorbitol, sucrose, calcium carbonate, sterile water, xanthan [Porcine circovirus type 1 (PCV1) is present in Rotarix. PCV-1 is not known to cause disease in humans.]
Smallpox (Vaccinia) (ACAM2000)	03/2018	HEPES, 2% human serum albumin, 0.5 - 0.7% sodium chloride USP, 5% Mannitol USP, neomycin, polymyxin B, 50% Glycerin USP, 0.25% phenol USP
Td (Tenivac)	11/2019	aluminum phosphate, formaldehyde, sodium chloride
Td (TDVAX)	09/2018	aluminum phosphate, formaldehyde, thimerosal
Tdap (Adacel)	12/2020	aluminum phosphate, formaldehyde, 2-phenoxyethanol, glutaraldehyde
Tdap (Boostrix)	09/2020	formaldehyde, aluminum hydroxide, sodium chloride, polysorbate 80
Typhoid (Typhim Vi)	03/2020	formaldehyde, phenol, polydimethylsiloxane, disodium phosphate, monosodium phosphate, sodium chloride
Typhoid (Vivotif Ty21a)	9/2013	sucrose, ascorbic acid, amino acids, lactose, magnesium stearate, gelatin
Varicella (Varivax) Frozen	01/2021[b]	sucrose, hydrolyzed gelatin, sodium chloride, monosodium L-glutamate, sodium phosphate dibasic, potassium phosphate monobasic, potassium chloride, MRC-5 human diploid cells including DNA & protein, sodium phosphate monobasic, EDTA, neomycin, fetal bovine serum
Yellow Fever (YF-Vax)	2/2019	sorbitol, gelatin, sodium chloride
Zoster (Shingles) (Shingrix)	01/2021[b]	sucrose, sodium chloride, dioleoyl phosphatidylcholine (DOPC), 3-O-desacl-4'monophosphoryl lipid A (MPL), QS-21 (a saponin purified from plant extract Quillaja saponaria Molina), potassium dihydrogen phosphate, cholesterol, sodium dihydrogen phosphate dihydrate, disodium phosphate anhydrous, dipotassium phosphate, polysorbate 80, host cell protein and DNA

C.J. ZINGLE

[Source: https://www.cdc.gov/vaccines/pubs/pinkbook/downloads/appendices/b/excipient-table-2.pdf?fbclid=IwAR0PYyTeX3DrTZ8U-Zf-hweoYnYw4sfMOXyXab41qDX9CO4qesm9QQXwhjY]

COVID-19 VACCINE INGREDIENTS

What Ingredients are in the COVID-19 Vaccines?

Many people are curious to know what the ingredients are for the three currently available COVID-19 vaccines in the US.

Here is a breakdown of the three COVID vaccines and their ingredients:

- **Pfizer Vaccine:** The full list of ingredients for the Pfizer vaccine is: mRNA, lipids ((4-hydroxybutyl)azanediyl)bis(hexane-6,1-diyl)bis(2-hexyldecanoate), 2 [(polyethylene glycol)-2000]-N,N-ditetradecylacetamide, 1,2-Distearoyl-sn-glycero-3-phosphocholine, and cholesterol), potassium chloride, monobasic potassium phosphate, sodium chloride, dibasic sodium phosphate dihydrate, and sucrose. **The Pfizer vaccine does not contain eggs, preservatives, or latex.**

- **Moderna Vaccine:** The full list of ingredients for the Moderna vaccine is: Messenger ribonucleic acid (mRNA), lipids (SM-102, polyethylene glycol [PEG] 2000 dimyristoyl glycerol [DMG], cholesterol, and 1,2-distearoyl-sn-glycero-3-phosphocholine [DSPC]), tromethamine,tromethamine hydrochloride, acetic acid, sodium acetate trihydrate, and sucrose. **The Moderna vaccine does not contain eggs, preservatives, or latex.**

- **Johnson & Johnson Vaccine:** The full list of ingredients for the Johnson & Johnson vaccine is: Recombinant, replication-incompetent adenovirus type 26 expressing the SARS-CoV-2 spike protein, citric acid monohydrate, trisodium citrate dihydrate, ethanol, 2 hydroxypropyl-β-cyclodextrin (HBCD), polysorbate-80, sodium chloride. **The Johnson & Johnson vaccine does not contain eggs, preservatives, or latex.**

(Source: What is the Full List of the COVID-19 Vaccine Ingredients? (ct.gov))

VACCINE DETOXIFICATION PROTOCOL

Vaccine Detoxification Protocol

The top 6 detoxing agents I recommend to detox and protect against shedding. (My reasoning will be explained below):

1. Zeoboost (Zeolite Powder)
2. Boron/Borax
3. Star Anise/Fennel
4. Chlorine Dioxide Solution (CDS)/MMS
5. NAC/Glutathione
6. Violet Ozone Ray High-Frequency Device

Zeoboost (Zeolite Powder) (Also helps cure cancer, autoimmune, autism, psoriasis, & more): To Detox The Heavy Metals

90 Day Zeolite Detox Instructions:

2 teaspoons of Zeoboost (Zeolite Powder) mixed in 16 oz of water 3 times a day or 3 teaspoons of Zeoboost (Zeolite Powder) mixed in 16 oz of water 2 times a day. I recommend starting with the 2 teaspoons and working your way up to the 3 teaspoons while your body adjusts. The powder does not have a taste so you will not need to worry about this. It is best to mix with water, to avoid the powder binding to anything prior to entering your body. You will follow this regiment for 90 days straight. You may notice some detox symptoms that may occur such as headaches and not being able to sleep within the first couple weeks of taking it. This is normal. If you experience sharp and/or uncomfortable pain, I would switch to a lower dose of only 1 teaspoon 3 times a day or less. Make sure NOT to handle the powder with metal. The powder binds to metal so DO NOT put in a metal container and make sure to use either plastic or glass. It is recommended that because Zeoboost is a binder, make sure to take it by itself and leave a 1-hour window between taking the Zeoboost and food/medication/supplements.

After the 90 days, you can cycle off of the Zeoboost for a week or two, and then take daily maintenance doses of 2 teaspoons a day mixed in 16oz of water. It is best to continue taking Zeolite due to all the toxins we are still being exposed to in our air, food, and water, currently.

Note: 1 jar of Zeoboost (90g) lasts about 7 days so if you would like to do the 90-day detox, you will need about 15 jars total. You should notice a difference after 1 jar. You do not have to do the full 90 days consecutively, it is best to start as soon as possible and if there are gaps in between, this will not have any impact on your detox. Zeoboost is what I used on my own personal journey, so I would highly recommend this brand. I also highly recommend Heiltropfen Brand. Please see conversions below to know how many jars will be needed to complete the 90-day detox. Both brands are highly recommended and I have used both.

90 Day Detox - Zeolite Powder Options:

- **15 Total Jars = Zeoboost (90g per jar)**
  Purchase Here: https://form.jotform.com/Zinglepathy_Rx/detox-order-form

- **3 Total Jars = Heiltropfen Zeolite 1LB (454g per jar)**
  Purchase Here:https://form.jotform.com/Zinglepathy_Rx/detox-order-form

- **6 Total Jars = Heiltropfen Zeolite 0.55LB (250g per jar)**
Purchase Here:https://form.jotform.com/Zinglepathy_Rx/detox-order-form

Zeolite Cautions:

- Taking too much zeolite without drinking enough water may cause dehydration and constipation so make sure you are well hydrated before starting a zeolite detox. To help prevent constipation, increase your fiber intake or supplement with magnesium.

- If you have major kidney problems, be cautious about your water intake and take minimum doses of zeolite.

- If you take more than 10g of zeolite powder per day over a very long period of time it may cause some loss of nutrition.

- DO NOT take iodine within 30 minutes of taking Zeolite

- DO NOT take zeolite at the same time as oil-based supplements, i.e. evening primrose oil or fish oil, as zeolite absorbs oil. Make sure to take these supplements at a separate time of day.

- DO NOT take zeolite at the same time as probiotics, as zeolite is antimicrobial.

- DO NOT take zeolite powder while you are taking a medication containing heavy metals, such as lithium, or containing platinum, which is found in some cancer medications. Instead, take zeolite after stopping the medication to help rid your body of the heavy metals.

- If you are having chemotherapy or radiation therapy, take zeolite before, between and after treatments but NOT during treatments.

Boron Tablets/Borax (also known to cure arthritis): To Detox The Nanotechnology

I personally have followed the Borax protocol. You can also purchase Boron tablets. I would also recommend taking Borax baths. Tablets can be purchased online or in store. Please follow the usage instructions on the bottle for the Boron Tablets, because products may vary. Borax powder can be found in the laundry aisle of pretty much any grocery store or store selling laundry detergent items.

Borax Protocol Instructions:

BORON MINERAL: ONLY known nanobot replication inhibitor.

You can take Borax OR Boron Tablets but do not take both. Follow instructions for each below:

Borax Detox (20 Mule Team Borax): Drink 1 pinch (1/16 teaspoon) in 1 pint of filtered water once a day. Build up to 3 times a day over time.

- Week 1 & 2: 1 pinch once daily.
- Week 3 & 4: 1 pinch twice daily.
- Week 5+: 1 pinch 3 times a day.

OR

Boron Tablets:

- Week 1 & 2: 3mg of Boron
- Week 3 & 4: 3mg in the morning & 3mg in the evening
- Week 5 & 6: 3mg in the morning, 3mg midday, & 3mg in the evening
- Week 7+: 6mg in the morning & 6mg in the evening

MAKE SURE TO LISTEN TO YOUR BODY ONCE YOU START INCREASING THE DOSE.

BORAX DETOX BATH:

1 Cup Baking Soda

1 Cup Epsom Salt

1 Cup 20 Mule Team Borax

1 Cup Pink Himalayan Sea Salt (NEVER use white depleted-minerals table salt for any reason)

SOAK AS LONG AS YOU CAN

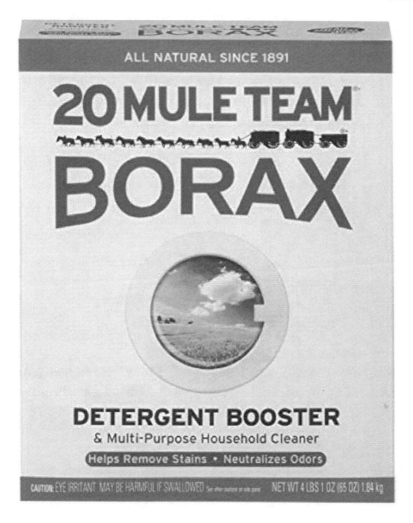

This mineral is intentionally depleted from the agricultural process.

Boron Benefits:

- Cures Arthritis
- Hormone Balance
- Decalcify Pineal Gland
- Improved Cell Function
- Improved Wound Healing
- Absorption of Minerals
- Encourages Proper pH: Cancer cannot live in an alkaline environment.
- Healthy Blood Sugar
- Detoxifies The Liver

- Helps The Heart

CANDIDA is an always-present fungus in the human body, there to help decompose the body after death. Taking a lot of antibiotics can cause candida overgrowth. Many suffer from it's overgrowth. Common Candida overgrowth symptoms include:

- Fatigue
- Brain Fog
- Digestive Issues
- Sinus Infections
- Thrush
- Joint Pain
- Depression
- Urinary Tract Infections
- Recurring Yeast Infection
- Other Fungal Infections

BORAX detoxes Fluoride from your body and brain. It raises your pH level from acid to alkaline. Cancer/Candida/Fungus/Nanobots cannot survive in a high alkaline pH environment.

Purchase Boron Tablets Here: https://form.jotform.com/Zinglepathy_Rx/detox-order-form

Star Anise and/or Fennel (Also known to help treat Autism): These are also an excellent source of shikimate or shikimic acid (which is known to neutralize the spike protein)

1 full dropper under tongue and swallow 3 times daily. **For at least 90 days.**

WHY IS SHIKIMIC ACID IMPORTANT TO US?

Shikimic acid offers antiplatelet-aggregating activity, suggesting it helps halt blood clots.

That study found that **pine needles provide about two-thirds the shikimic acid of star anise herb:**

Masson pine needles = **5.71%** shikimic acid
Star anise = **8.95%** shikimic acid

That pine needle tea **(all the safe pine tree varieties) offers a solution to stop the vascular damage** (and is possibly an antidote against the effects of c o v i d vaccine transmission) is really good news!

Fennel is a plant in the carrot and celery family. It tastes sweet and licoricey and is also highly aromatic. Fennel has been used as medicine for thousands of years.

The active ingredient in fennel seeds is shikimic acid.

Star anise contains many medicinal compounds that contribute to its long list of health benefits.

As concerns continue to mount over the threat to global health, the demand for star anise is on the rise.

(Source: https://www.researchgate.net/ *publication/277348748_Content_Analysis_of_Shikimic_Acid_in_the_Masson_Pine_Needles_and_Antiplatelet-aggregating_Activity)*

(Source: https://www.naturalnews.com/2021-05-07-salk-institute-reveals-the-covid-spike-protein-causing-deadly-blood-clots.html)

(Source: https://www.researchgate.net/publication/305639160_Anti-platelet_and_anti- *thrombogenic_effects_of_shikimic_acid_in_sedentary_population)*

(Source: https://draxe.com/nutrition/star-anise/)

Purchase Here:
https://form.jotform.com/Zinglepathy_Rx/detox-order-form

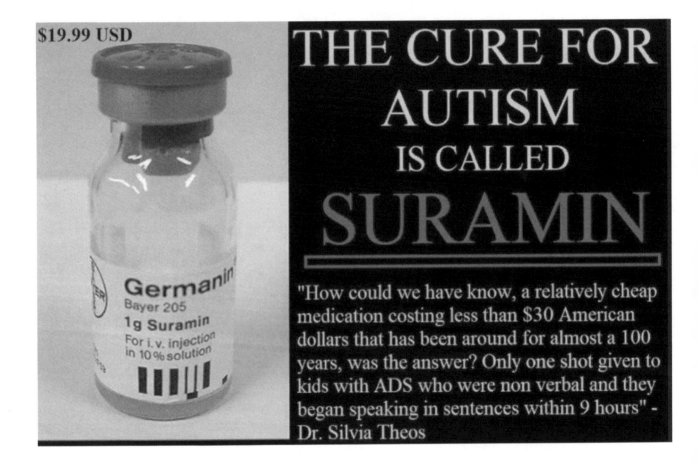

Chlorine Dioxide (CDS) or Miracle Mineral Supplement (MMS) Chlorine dioxide neutralizes and eliminates the spikes (also known to cure cancer & AIDS/HIV):

Vitamin C neutralizes this substance so in other words, do NOT use the chlorine dioxide protocol at the same time as any substance which has Vitamin C, or any other antioxidant, including immune builders. Wait at least a couple of days after discontinuing these treatments before starting the chlorine dioxide treatment.

Drink on an empty stomach. Mix 12 drops of part A with 12 drops of part B in 16oz of water. Allow to activate for 1 minute. Wait 30min to eat after drinking. After you have eaten wait 45min to begin drink again.

Days 1-2: Drink 2oz every hour
Days 3-4: Drink 4oz every hour
Days 5-6: Drink 6oz every hour
Days 7-Beyond: Drink 8oz every hour - Do this for as long as issues/symptoms persist & then once issues are gone switch to maintenance 2 drinks a day morning & evening.

Purchase Here: https://form.jotform.com/Zinglepathy_Rx/detox-order-form

MMS Background Information: The Miracle Mineral Supplement (educate-yourself.org)

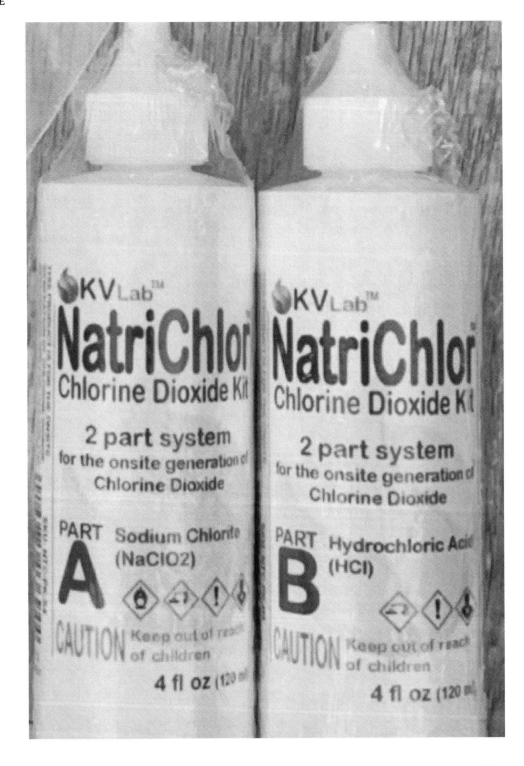

NAC (N-acetyl cysteine): NAC/Glutathione neutralizes the Graphene Oxide, as well as spikes to some extent.

NAC (N-acetyl cysteine) (accelerates detoxification and is considered a producer of the super detoxifier glutathione in the body) Dosage: 1200-2400 mg per day on an empty stomach. NAC is recommended to detoxify graphene oxide and SM-102. NAC is tough to find after the FDA recently made it illegal to purchase over the counter in the USA. Take NAC daily for at least 90 days. NAC can be taken daily for extended period of time. There are no known health damages caused by taking it daily for extended periods of time.

Purchase Here : https://form.jotform.com/Zinglepathy_Rx/detox-order-form

Violet Ozone Ray High-Frequency Device

Violet Ray is an electrotherapy medical appliance used during the early 20th century. Nikola Tesla invented the basic construction of the Violet Ray prior to 1900. Tesla's coil is really an electrical resonant transformer circuit. Using a disruptive discharge coil with an interrupter that applies a low current, a high voltage, with a high frequency. Tesla introduced the first prototypes at the World's Columbian Exposition in 1893.

The Violet Ray appliance is a high-frequency, high voltage, low current source of static electricity. It can be applied to any part of the body. The Violet Ray brings a vigorous surge of rich, warm blood to any part of the body. Thereby it washes away the sediment of a disease, then strengthens and nourishes the tissues, and gives vigor and vitality to any part of the body that is treated.

SCIENTIFICALLY ACCEPTED EFFECTS OF VIOLET RAYS:

1—Cause cells to absorb more oxygen.

2—Speed up burning of oxygen.

3—Increase elimination of waste.

4—Restore cells to health.

5—Increase blood supply in given area.

6—Stimulate secretions of glands.

7—Raise body heat without temperature.

8—Destroy germs.

9—Soothe the nerves; build nerve tissue.

10—Remove dead tissue and adhesions.

11—Lower blood pressure.

12—Promote normal growth.

AILMENTS SUCCESSFULLY TREATED WITH VIOLET RAYS:

- Asthma

- Boils

- Brain Fag

- Bronchitis

- Catarrh

- Colds in Head

- Colds in Lungs

- Constipation

- Dandruff

- Deafness

- Dyspepsia

- Earache

- Eczema

- Eye Disease

- Falling Hair

- Hay Fever

- Headaches

- Insomnia

- Influenza

- Goiter

- Lumbago

- Nervousness

- Neuralgia

- Neuritis

- Obesity

- Pimples

- Pneumonia

- Prostate Gland

- Rheumatism

- Scars

- Skin Diseases

- Sore Throat

- Sprains

- Stiff Neck or joints

- Tonsilitis Ulcers

Instructions: Please make sure to read the handbook included with the device for the safety precautions and use instructions prior to using the device. Follow the instructions for use in the handbook based on the symptoms you are experiencing post-vaccine.

Violet Ray Precautions - Please Read Before Purchasing:

The device should not be used near metal plates and pins. The device should not be used near metal jewelry, so please remove any jewelry in the areas you will be treating. This device has a high-frequency and cannot be used if you have a pacemaker or have an electronic hearing implant. The Violet Ray should not be used if you have drank any alcohol. Fatal complications can occur if alcohol is in your blood. If you have a heart murmur or heart disease, the Violet Ray should be used from the back only. Do not move the Violet Ray directly over the heart.

Purchase Here: https://form.jotform.com/Zinglepathy_Rx/detox-order-form

ADDITIONAL DETOXING REMEDIES & PROTECTION

Additional Detoxing Remedies & Protection:

Here is a list of additional remedies to prevent damage from the spike protein and derivatives due to injection and to protect from spike protein shedding of those who have been vaccinated:

- **Alpha Lipoic Acid (ALA):** An antioxidant to strengthen the cardiovascular system and keep it clear. A potent promoter of glutathione. Has shown success in stroke recovery, HIV and AIDS, heavy metal toxicity and detoxification support as well as many other treatment abilities.

- **Andrographis:** Helps prevent clogging of arteries and second heart attack after angioplasty. Credited for stopping the virulent Indian Flu epidemic in 1919. Anti-inflammatory and antibiotic action, and works especially well in combination with Vitamin C, bioflavonoids, and echinacea.

- **Arjuna:** An ayurvedic heart tonic effective for angina pain, arrhythmia, and congestive heart failure. High antioxidants in the tannins and flavones prevent oxidative damage linked to heart disease.

- **Astragulus:** A strong immune enhancer, a vasodilator that helps lower blood pressure and increase circulation. Keeps nasal-passage linings from lettings in rhinoviruses. Improves circulation after heart attack, helps prevent second heart attack. Very important if heart problem related to a virus develops.

- **Bromelain:** Anti-inflammatory and clot inhibitor for fragile veins. Increases the breakdown of fibrin, which forms around the inflamed area, blocking the blood and lymphatic vessels.

- **Glucosamine/Chondroitin:** Anti-thrombogenic, anti-coagulant.

- **Grape Seed Extract (GSE):** 50x stronger than Vitamin E, 20x stronger than Vitamin C, and they are one of the few antioxidants that readily cross the blood-brain barrier to protect brain cells and aid memory.

- **Hawthorn (In heart emergency, one half dropperful every 15 minutes):** Bioflavonoid-rich, and adept at counteracting the damaging effects of free radicals on the cardiovascular system. Gentle but powerful. Improves blood flow to the heart and cardiac enzymes, which measure damage to heart muscle. Relaxes muscles surrounding arteries. Lowers both blood pressure and cholesterol levels. Helps the liver convert LDL into HDL. Helps preserve blood-vessel integrity after transient ischemic attacks (TIAs) (mini-strokes).

- **Quercetin** (500-1000 mg, twice daily)

- **Raw Garlic Cloves** (Eat 3 cloves of garlic every morning or take a teaspoon of garlic oil. Can also be used by mixing crushed garlic in a little cold water and drink the mixture immediately. Garlic can also prevent against the virus and is a very stringent parasite removing substance.)

- **Lypospheric Vitamin C** (30ml, twice daily)

- **Coated Silver** (1-6 drops per day, depending on degree of exposure) (Coated silver blocks the sulfur-bearing protein on the spikes from entering the cell. Sulfur-rich amino acids on the spike protein interact with silver causing them to fold incorrectly).

- **Zinc** (30-80mg per day depending on immunological pressure)

- **Vitamin D3** (10,000 IU's per day)

- **Iodine** (dosage depends on brand, more is not better. Iodine is a product you have to start with small dosages and build up over time.)

- **MRM, Cardio Chelate with EDTA:** Cardio Chelate™ is a combination of nutrients that are designed to support cardiovascular health and promote healthy blood flow. Ethylene-Diamine-Tetra-Acetic Acid (EDTA) is a chelating agent with antioxidant properties and can bind to free-flowing metal ions in the bloodstream, forming a chemical bond that can facilitate the removal of these complexes. This can help suppress the development of damaging free radicals and any chain reaction that they might cause. While EDTA can remove toxic metals and abnormally metabolized minerals from the body, its effects may be enhanced by including Vitamin C, Methyl-Sulfonyl-Methane (MSM), and N-Acetyl-Cysteine (NAC). These nutrients are vital for supporting the liver and other tissues during the detoxification process. MSM and NAC are precursors to glutathione; a powerful free radical scavenger involved in the liver's detoxifying enzyme system. Vitamin C is a proven antioxidant and has been shown to support cardiovascular health.

- **Pyrroloquinoline quinone (PQQ)** (20-40 mg per day)

Shikimate Main Sources:

- **Fennel and/or Star Anise:** These are also an excellent source of shikimate or shikimic acid (which is known to neutralize the spike protein)

Purchase Here: https://form.jotform.com/Zinglepathy_Rx/detox-order-form

- **Pine Needle Tea for shikimic acid or shikimate** (There are toxic pine needles, be careful! When drinking pine needle tea, drink the oil/resin that accumulates too! Shikimate, shikimic acid and their derivatives possess: cancer fighting, antiviral, antimicrobial, anticoagulant and antithrombotic properties.)
  - YouTube: (462) White Pine - Identification and Uses - YouTube
  - PINE TEA: Possible Antidote for Spike Protein Transmission – Ariyana Love (wordpress.com)
- **C60** (1-3 droppersfull per day): One of the issues we are seeing with those who have been injected is disturbances in their energetic field (magnetism) and hot spots of inflammation. C60 is a rich-source of electrons and acts like a fire extinguisher to inflammation and simultaneously (because it bio-distributes throughout the body) drives a normalization of electron flow throughout the body. C60 is recommended to neutralize spike protein, detoxify graphene oxide and SM-102.
- **Activated Charcoal (2-4 capsules a day):** Activated Charcoal is the pre-eminent detoxifier and when taken on an empty stomach, works its way down into the intestines and activates a blood purification process known as "interstitial dialysis". Activated charcoal should not be taken over long periods of time. Take for 5 days, at most, at any given time.

- **Citrus fruit** (especially blood oranges, due to their high hesperidin content — hesperidin is a chalcone like quercetin that deactivates spike protein)

- **Peppermint** (very high in hesperidin)

- **Wheatgrass and Wheatgrass Juice** (blades are high in shikimate)

Superherbs to help disable the spike protein:

- **Schizandra Berry** (high in shikimate)

- **Triphala formulations**: In Sanskrit, the word Triphala means "three fruits": a combination of Indian gooseberry (Emblica officinalis), black myrobalan (Terminalia chebula) and belleric myrobalan (Terminalia belerica). The terminalia fruits are rich in shikimate.

- **St. John's Wort** (shikimate is found throughout the entire plant and in the flowers)

- **Feverfew** (leaves and flowers are rich in shikimate)
- **Comfrey Leaf** (rich in shikimate)
- **Gingko Biloba Leaf** (rich in shikimate)
- **Giant Hyssop or Horsemint** (Agastache urtifolia) (rich in shikimate)
- **Liquid Ambar (Sweet Gum tree):** Rich in shikimate.
- **Olive Leaf Extract:** Prevents damage from the spike protein. Olive Leaf Extract attenuates inflammatory activation and DNA damage in human arterial endothelial cells.

BLOCKING VS. NEUTRALIZING THE SPIKE PROTEIN

Blocking vs. Neutralizing The Spike Protein:

- **Quercetin or Hydroxychloroquine (HCQ):** Quercetin works like HCQ. One of its mechanisms of action is that it blocks the 'virus' (with spikes around it) from attaching. These two supplements will help with spike protein damage and apply to most organs of the body but not all.

- **Ivermectin(IVM):** Ivermectin blocks spike proteins from attaching to the cell membrane. *(Alternative is Neem Oil and "Sweet Wormwood" (Artemisia Annua) – Being used in other countries and has been used to treat Malaria in the past.)*

- **Dandelion Leaf:** Dandelion Leaf Extract blocks spike proteins from attaching to cell membrane.

- **Chlorine Dioxide (CDS)** or Miracle Mineral Supplement (MMS) Chlorine dioxide neutralizes and eliminates the spikes.

Between a blocker (HCQ, Quercetin, Ivermectin, Dandelion, etc), and a neutralizer (CDS/MMS, Ozone, NAC), I prefer a neutralizer because it eliminates the spikes rather than only blocking them. I suggest alternating this with NAC in case there is Graphene Oxide transmission. I worry that the blocked spikes will continue to circulate and reach the brain and cause all sorts of mental illnesses (Dr. Malone, Bahkdi, Tenpenny, Mikovits). Most people prefer Chlorine Dioxide (CDS) to de-magnetize the body and NAC along with star anise and/or fennel or white pine tea. Make sure to stock up as the FDA is trying to ban some herbs and seeds and supplements.

- Chlorine dioxide (CDS) neutralizes the spikes.
- NAC or Glutathione neutralizes the Graphene Oxide, as well as spikes to some extent.
- For protection, I will alternate use of Chlorine dioxide and NAC.

We now have evidence of the latest injections containing: mRNA, spike protein, graphene oxide, SM-102, and numerous other potentially toxic substances.

Source: https://www.planet-today.com/2021/09/american-scientists-confirm-toxic.html#gsc.tab=0

Home Recipe For Hydroxychloroquine (HCQ)

What is Hydroxychloroquine exactly?

It is nothing but Quinine. Something that anyone can make at home... and something that is being manufactured each and every day in the form of something we have all seen at the grocery and liquor stores. This drug is being used to treat the Covid-19 virus.

Quinine has many uses and applications. It is analgesic, anesthetic, anti-arrhythmic, anti-bacterial, anti-malarial, anti-microbial, anti-parasitic, antipyretic, antiseptic, antispasmodic, antiviral, astringent, bactericide, cytotoxic, febrifuge, fungicide, insecticide, nervine, and much more.

If you ever feel a chest cold coming on or just feel like crap... make your own quinine. It is made out of the peelings of grapefruits and lemons but especially grapefruits.

Here is all you need to make your own quinine:

- Take the rind of 2-3 lemons, 2-3 grapefruits
- Take the peel ONLY and cover it with water about 3 inches above the peels.
- Put a glass lid on the pot, and let it simmer for about 2 hours.
- Do not take the lid off of the pot until it cools completely as this will allow the quinine to escape in the steam.
- Sweeten the tea with honey since it will be bitter. Take 1 tablespoon every couple of hours to bring up the phlegm from your lungs. Discontinue as soon as you get better.

WHAT WE CURRENTLY KNOW ABOUT GRAPHENE OXIDE (GO)

What we currently know about Graphene Oxide (GO):

- Graphene Oxide fibers are in plastic masks.
- Graphene Oxide blocks detoxification in the body by blocking glutathione.
- Graphene Oxide creates thromboses.
- Graphene Oxide causes blood clots.
- Graphene Oxide fibers are on PCR test swabs.
- Graphene Oxide is in all Covid-19 vaccines.
- Graphene Oxide disrupts the immune system.
- Graphene Oxide can trigger a cytokine storm.
- Graphene Oxide toxicity can instigate pneumonia.
- Graphene Oxide creates a metallic taste in the mouth.
- Graphene Oxide causes inflammation of the mucous membranes.
- Graphene Oxide produces a loss in the sense of taste and smell.
- Graphene Oxide is magnetic (especially at the injection site.)
- Graphene Oxide may be activated by 5G frequencies.
- Graphene Oxide was already included as an adjuvant in the flu shots in 2019.
- Graphene Oxide passes thru the blood-brain barrier.
- Graphene Oxide can act as a solo trigger for most COVID symptoms.

*****This is not a VIRUS or spike protein, but a chemical warfare agent.*****

Vaccine Patient Blood Samples:

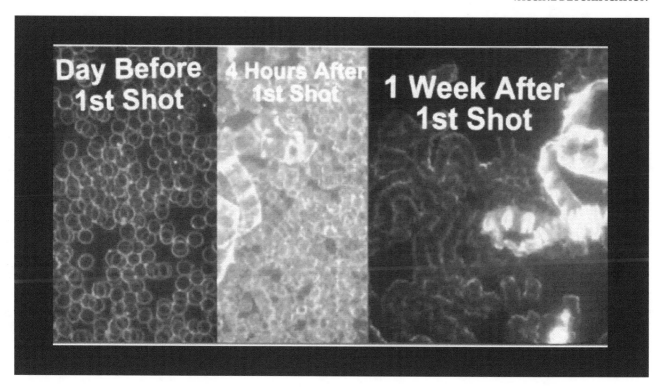

Vaccine Sample Compared With Graphene:

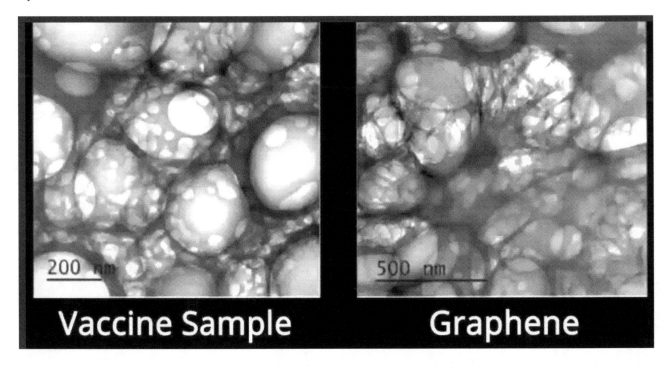

Vaccine Sample / Graphene

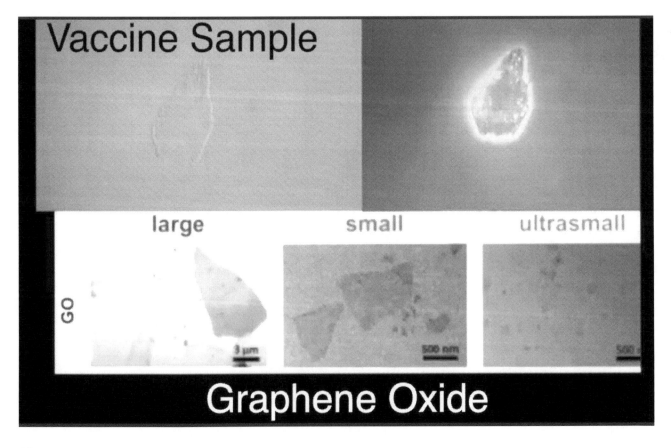

Vaccine Sample

GO — large / small / ultrasmall

Graphene Oxide

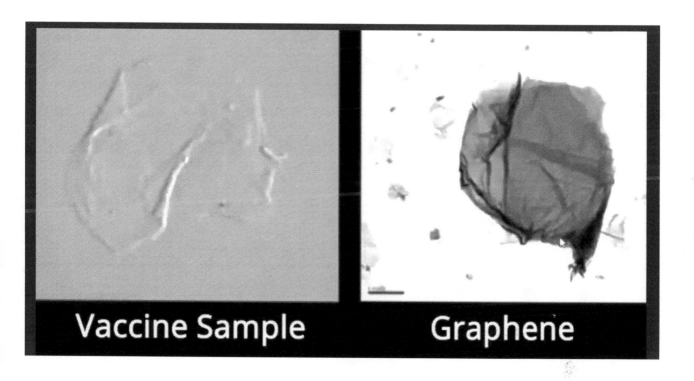

Vaccine Sample   Graphene

USEFUL REMEDIES FOR TREATING & PREVENTING VIRUS

Useful Remedies For Treating & Preventing Virus:

Click This Link To Visit My Other Blog Post:

COVID-19 Virus: Prevention & Infection Remedies List Post - www. zinglepathy.com

FURTHER RESEARCH - SCIENTIFIC STUDIES RELATING TO VACCINE INJURIES

Click Here For A Compiled List Of Over 200+ Scientific Studies Proving Correlation Between Vaccine Injury And Their Association In Major Health Disorders And Illnesses:

Maybe It's 'Genetics' OR Maybe It's a VACCINE INJURY - A Compilation Of Historical Vaccine Injury Studies (zinglepathy.com)

Frequently reported Neurological adverse effects

Adverse effect		Vaccines
Demyelination disease	Multiple sclerosis (MS)	Hepatitis B vaccine [50]
	Acute disseminated encephalomyelitis (ADEM)	Human papillomavirus vaccine [51]
	Transverse myelitis	Influenza vaccine
	Optic neuritis	Rabies vaccine [52]
		Yellow fever vaccine [53]
Guillain-Barré syndrome (GBS)		Influenza vaccine [54]
		Oral polio vaccine
		Tetanus vaccines [55]
Encephalopathy		Whole-cell pertussis vaccine [56]
		Influenza Vaccine
Seizure		Diphtheria, tetanus toxoids and whole-cell pertussis vaccine (DTP)
		Measles, mumps, and rubella vaccine (MMR) [9]
Autism		MMR [57], [a]

[a]The original manuscript had been withdrawn.

AUTOIMMUNE DISEASE

VACCINE

Measles, mumps, nubela (MMR)

Yellow fever

Bacillus Calmette-Guerin (BCG)

Hepatitis B virus (HBV)

Human Papilloma Virus (HPV)

Influenza

Meningococcal

Pneumococcal

Diphtheria-Tetanus-Pertussis (dTP)

Varicella

Small Pox

Arthrex

H1N1 Influenza

Rotavirus

idiopathic thrombocytopenic purpura
Arthralgia/Arthritis including rheumatoid arthritis
Neurologic disease- related to yellow fever
Dermatomyositis
Takayasu's arteritis
Optic neuritis
Guillain Barre Syndrome (GBS)
Myelitis
Multiple Sclerosis
Systemic lupus erythematosus (SLE)
Antiphospholipid syndrome (APS)
Myopathy/Myositis
Acute disseminated encephalomyelitis
Transverse Myelitis
Pancreatitis
Postural Orthostatic tachycardia syndrome (POT)
Primary Ovarian Failure (POF)
Autoimmune hepatitis
Vasculitis
Henoch-Schonlein purpura (HSP)
Bullous Pemphigiod
Narcolepsy
Celiac disease
Polymyalgia rheumatica
Fibromyalgia/Chronic Fatigue syndrome

@cjzingle

83

Vaccine Injury is nothing new... it's just rarely talked about...

Vaccine injuries are more common than most people know.

This post will include the following sections below:

- Vaccination as Contamination
- Aseptic Meningitis and the MMR
- Vaccinations and Leukemia/Lymphomas
- Vaccines and Chromosome Changes Leading to Mutations
- Vaccines and Autoimmunity
- Vaccinations and Diabetes
- Other Articles Linking Diabetes to Vaccines
- Vaccines and Nervous System Changes
- Vaccines and Demyelination
- Vaccinations and Seizures
- Vaccines and Brain Swelling
- Vaccines and Neurological Damage
- Vaccinations and Unexplained Diseases
- Vaccines and Metabolism
- Vaccines and Skin Disorders
- The Polio Vaccine and Cancer
- Vaccinations and Autism
- Resolving and Reversing Vaccine Injury

FINAL NOTES

Final Notes

An overly acidic environment will create the perfect breeding ground for the contents in the vaccine to react within your body and therefore, an alkaline diet would be best. Below is a table foods… try to consume alkaline foods (at the top) and limit/avoid acidic foods (at the bottom), if possible.

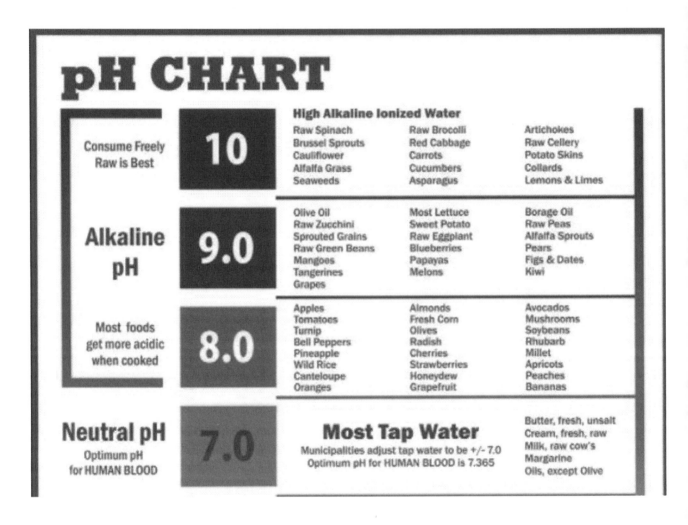

It takes 20 parts
of ALKALINITY
to neutralize
1 part ACIDITY
in the body

Acidic
pH

Consume
sparingly
or never

6.0			
	Milk, Yogurt	Fruit Juices	Cooked Spinach
	Most Grains	Soy Milk, Goat's Milk	Coconut
	Eggs	Fish	Tea
	Kidney Beans	Lima Beans	Plums
	Processed Juices	Rye Bread	Spelt
	Brown Rice	Cocoa	Rice & Almond Milk
	Sprouted Wheat Bread	Oats	Liver
	Oysters	Cold Water Fish	Salmon, Tuna

5.0			
	Cooked Beans	Chicken & Turkey	Beer
	Sugar	Canned Fruit	White Rice
	Potatoes w/o Skins	Pinto Beans	Navy Beans
	Garbanzos	Lentils	Black Beans
	Butter, salted	Rice Cakes	Cooked Corn
	Wheat Bran	Rhubarb	Molasses

4.0			
	Reverse Osmosis Water	Distilled & Purified Water	Most Bottled Water & Sports Drinks
	Coffee	White Bread	
	Pistachios	Beef	Blackberries
	Cranberries	Prunes	Sweetened Fruit Juices
	Wheat	Most Nuts	Tomato Sauce
	Popcorn	Peanuts	

3.0			
	Lamb	Pork	Wine
	Shellfish	Pastries	Cheese
	Goat Cheese	Soda	Black Tea
	Pasta	Pickles	Stress
	Worry	Lack of Sleep	Overwork
	Tobacco Smoke	Chocolate	Vinegar
	Sweet'N Low	Equal	Aspartame
	NutraSweet	Processed Food	Microwaved Foods

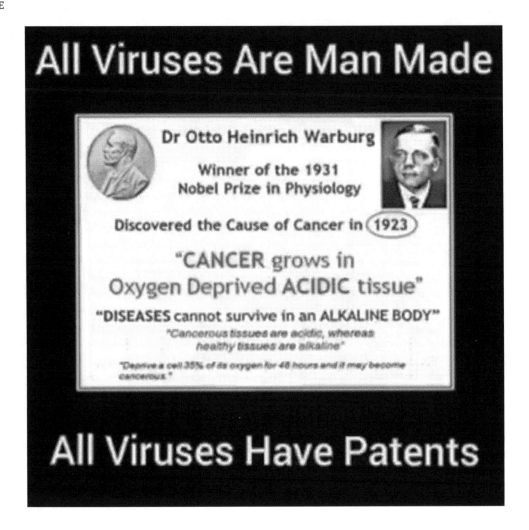

Lastly, remember that our journey here is one for soul growth and expansion... and this situation is part of the test and soul journey. In 2013, I had began suffering from many detrimental health symptoms and issues caused by the Gardasil HPV vaccine I had gotten in 2008 when I was 19. Beginning in 2013, I had been diagnosed with an autoimmune disease - Hashimoto's, endometriosis, deep depression, and eventually psoriasis...all triggered by a vaccine...and the symptoms got progressively worse with passing time. Prior to the vaccine I had ZERO of these health issues or symptoms. Looking back on it now, the health issues I gained due to the vaccine were the biggest part of my awakening and it truly helped to jumpstart my awakening journey. Without them and the vaccine, I would not be who and where I am today. It was a humbling experience that pushed me to look for answers both personally and inwardly, as well as externally. Prior to the vaccine I had taken my good health and life for granted... but the adversity I faced and the pain I suffered from after the vaccine was a huge wake up call for me that helped me to remember I should be grateful for what I have daily. It also helped me to rekindle my connection with God and my faith. Although it was a lot of suffering, it was the catalyst in my awakening... and I think everyone should keep this in mind. I wouldn't go back and change any part of what I went through because it all made me into the person I am today. I provided my personal story in the next section.

Remember to forgive yourself for the decisions you made before you knew any better... we've all been there and you are not alone. Forgiveness of self and others on our journey is one of the most important lessons to overcome and learn here. Use this time of healing to become closer to God/Source Creator (whatever you imagine them to be). Without full faith in God, you will not survive this test or journey or the times. Make sure to pray daily for healing, guidance, strength, and anything you need help with or need. Lastly, spend time in daily meditation imagining yourself healthy and happy.

Find yourself a Naturopathic Doctor near you to switch to... you can find one using this search:

https://naturopathic.org/search/custom.asp?id=5613

Always keep the faith and hope that everything happens and turns out for the best and for our highest good... I'm a firm believer that anything can be healed and resolved through God if we keep the faith and fully trust in God's plan for us and pray daily.

Please pass this protocol along to anyone who may need it and make sure to save somewhere for yourself!

MY VACCINE INJURY STORY

My Vaccine Injury Story

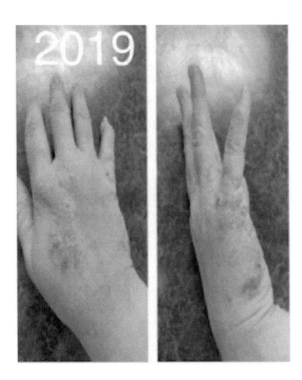
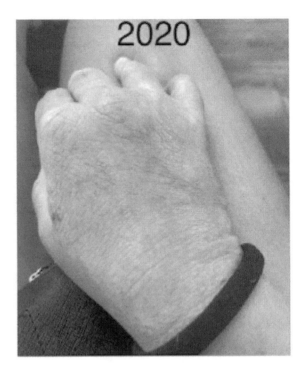

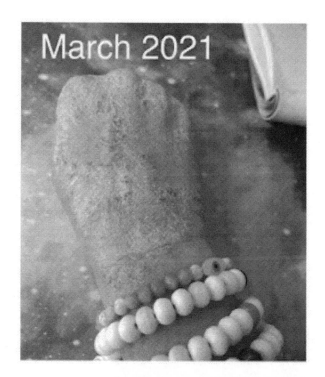

March 2021

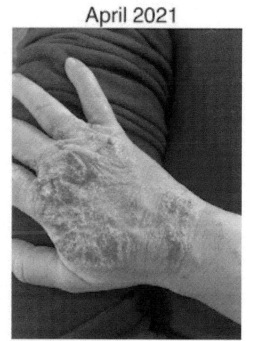

April 2021

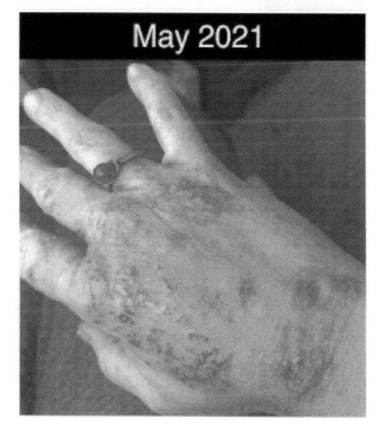

May 2021

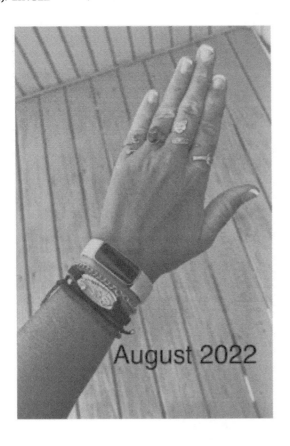

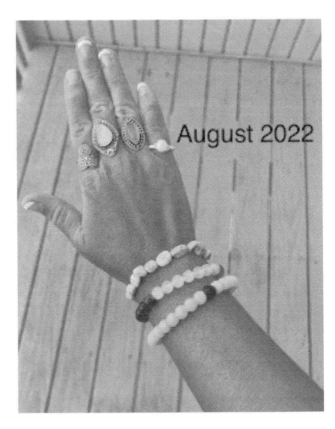

In 2013, I was diagnosed with Hashimoto's thyroiditis
(an autoimmune disease) and in summer 2018 I began developing a weird rash on my hand that was later diagnosed as psoriasis... the psoriasis was just another symptom that had stemmed from my autoimmune disease... since 2013 I went to many doctors to try and find a cure for my autoimmune and psoriasis and for many years I was given no answers and told I just had to deal with it... "try the elimination diet" they said... I tried the elimination diet and still nothing was resolved... I decided to become an advocate for myself and finally figure out the root cause of my health problems that seemed to get worse and worse with each passing year...

In July 2021 I stumbled on a product called "Zeoboost" (after trying everything under the sun and nothing working)... Zeoboost is a micronized Zeolite Clinoptilolite powder... after much research, I decided to try a 90 day detox using Zeoboost, taking 2 teaspoons of the powder mixed in 16oz of water three times a day. After about a week of following this regiment I noticed many of my symptoms began resolving... I no longer had extreme fatigue, my energy levels were much better and elevated, and my psoriasis began to clear from my hands... it took about 2 months for my psoriasis to completely clear and as time went on I noticed all the symptoms from my autoimmune began to resolve and reverse... today my hands are completely clear... which I am very grateful for.

Living with psoriasis, and especially when it is on your hands, was probably one of the most ongoing stressful situations I have ever experienced... in the winter I would hide my hands under winter gloves, while dreading the arrival of spring and summer (which had always been my favorite time of the year)... there was no easy way to cover and hide it during these months, and so I spent most of my time at home and went out only when I really needed to... people would see my hands and try their best to be polite about asking what was wrong with my hands... most people were genuinely concerned because they thought it looked extremely painful and they wanted to make sure it wasn't contagious poison ivy .

My journey reversing my autoimmune disease and psoriasis was the inspiration for my first book on detoxing... and it has helped many people this year with their own health issues.

Many people think that illness can be resolved and cured by adding pharmaceutical drugs to their bodies... but nothing is healed until we discover the ROOT CAUSE of the symptoms in the first place... pHARMa misses this part in the healing process. The drugs that are developed are tasked to mask and resolve the symptoms but the symptoms are there for a reason. The body is trying to notify us there is an underlying problem that must be dealt with... the body does not need addition of supplements and drugs, but the elimination of what is causing the health ailment in the first place...

CURES come when we DETOX the toxins in our bodies causing the underlying dis-ease.

Please share this story with whoever may need it... many people suffering from psoriasis and autoimmune diseases believe that their situation is completely hopeless... but I am evidence that it is not, and that it can truly be reversed and cured.

COVID-19 VACCINE INJURIES
I'VE PERSONALLY WITNESSED

Covid-19 Vaccine Injuries I've Personally Witnessed:

Here is a list and timeline of people I have seen impacted by these vaccines on a personal level. I have not included any personal information of the individuals due to keeping anonymity. This list was updated January 2023:

- 2021: Covid-19 vaccinated longtime family friend passed away due to blood clot in leg.

- March 2021: Bestfriend's brother gets a dead arm and numb left side of body after receiving the Covid-19 vaccine. Excruciating arm pain that he seeks medical attention for. Had to red shirt his junior year season playing Division 1 soccer due to pain and numbness on left side of body.

- April 2021: A boy I had graduated with was diagnosed with brain tumors suddenly, weeks after receiving covid-19 vaccine. Prior to the vaccines he was in good health and 2 weeks after receiving the vaccine, his wife noticed he seemed out of it and health began to decline. They did a bunch of diagnostic testing and found largely developed brain tumors. He passed away Fall 2022.

- 2021: Uncle develops arrhythmia from covid-19 vaccines.

- March 2022: Cousin in-law passed away suddenly at work from a swollen heart. He was only 29 years old and played D1 baseball. He was perfectly healthy prior to receiving the Covid-19 vaccines.

- May 2022: Aunt develops blood clot in her leg that needed to be emergency surgically removed.

- June 2022: A friend who was a long-time firefighter and was forced to get the Covid-19 vaccines for work, dies of a heart attack in his girlfriend's arms one night. The girlfriend is a longtime family friend.

- October 2022: Vaccinated Aunt passes away from blood clot complications of the vaccine.

These are just 8 different personal accounts of people I know who have been impacted by the Covid-19 vaccines... I am sure I am not the only one who has witnessed events like the above... the severity of damage that has occurred in such little time. Please continue to share these kinds of stories with others in order to help wake people up to the connections relating to the vaccines. There are many scientific health studies to be found, connecting the vaccine to these health impacts and deaths... but the media doesn't want you to know that. If you need help pulling the scientific studies for your own situation, I am well-versed in finding these studies and know exactly where to look. Please reach out to me via rx@zinglepathy.com .

None of this is 'just a coincidence'!

FURTHER READING

Further Reading:

1. **Behavioral Problems in Childhood: The Link to Vaccination**, By Viera Scheibner

2. **Bodily Matters: The Anti-Vaccination Movement in England 1853-1907**, By Nadja Durbach

3. **Changing The Course of Autism: A Scientific Approach for Parents and Physicians**, By Bryan Jepson

4. **Children With Starving Brains: A Medical Treatment Guide for Autism Spectrum Disorder**, By Jaquelyn Mccandless

5. **Confessions Of a Medical Heretic**, By Robert S. Mendelsohn

6. **Dangers Of Compulsory Immunizations: How to Avoid Them Legally,** By Tom Finn, Esq.

7. **Dissent In Medicine: Nine Doctors Speak Out**, By Robert S. Mendelsohn

8. **Don't Vaccinate Before You Educate**, By Mayer Eisenstein

9. **Dr. Mary's Monkey: How the Unsolved Murder of a Doctor, A Secret Laboratory in New Orleans and Cancer-Causing Monkey Viruses Are Linked To Lee Harvey Oswald, Assassination And Emerging Global Epidemics**, By Edward T. Haslam

10. **Emerging Viruses: Aids and Ebola: Nature, Accident or Intentional?** By Leonard Horowitz

11. **Every Second Child**, By Archie Kalokerinos

12. **Evidence Of Harm: Mercury in Vaccines and The Autism Epidemic: A Medical Controversy**, By David Kirby

13. **Fear Of the Invisible**, By Janine Roberts

14. **How To End the Autism Epidemic**, By J.B. Handley

15. **Fowl! Bird Flu: It's Not What You Think**, By Sherri Tenpenny

16. **The Immunization Decision: A Guide for Parents**, By Randall Neustaedter

17. **The Immunization Resource Guide: Where to Find Answers to All Your Questions About Childhood Vaccinations**, By Diane Rozario

18. **The Infant Survival Guide Protecting Your Baby from The Dangers of Crib**

FOLLOW ME HERE FOR
MORE UPDATES

C.J. ZINGLE

<u>Follow Me Here For More Updates</u>

Email: Rx@zinglepathy.com

Follow me on Truth Social & AnonUp for new insights and inspiration daily: @cjzingle

TikTok: @cjzingle

Instagram: @cjzingle

My Telegram Channel: https://t.me/xoanara

Personal Blog: Zinglepathy: Naturopathic Healing - https://www.zinglepathy.com/

My Online Store For Natural Remedies: https://form.jotform.com/Zinglepathy_Rx/detox-order-form

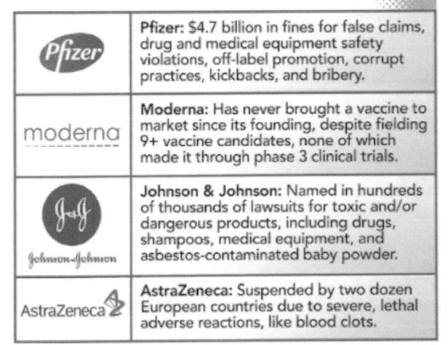

106

ABOUT THE AUTHOR

C.j. Zingle

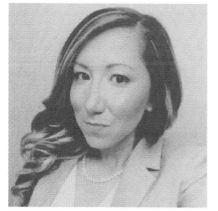

C.J. Zingle was born and raised in Philadelphia, Pennsylvania, USA. She pursued a degree in Chemistry from Mount St. Mary's University in Maryland, where she was granted a Softball Scholarship to play Division 1 Softball and Soccer. Upon graduating with a Chemistry undergraduate degree in 2011, she was asked to be the Assistant Coach for the Women's Softball program and helped coach The Mount for 3 seasons while pursuing her Master of Business Administration (M.B.A.) degree.

After completing her Master's degree, she pursued a diversified Scientific career in the Pharmaceutical industry from 2015-2020. A highly distinguished Pharmaceutical and CRO professional in Large Molecule Pharmaceutical R&D and manufacturing, with experience supporting biologics drug discovery, sample analysis, clinical and non-clinical method development, assay validation work, method transfer outsourcing projects, Quality Control analytical testing for raw materials for drug formulation and analytical testing for extended release (XR) and immediate release (IR) finished products, across all therapeutic areas spanning non-clinical studies to post-market clinical development in R&D and also experience in pharmaceutical drug formulation and manufacturing of finished products.

She has a comprehensive background in Biologics, including knowledge and experience in Anti-Drug Antibodies (ADA), Pharmacokinetics (PK) and Anti-Drug Neutralizing Antibodies(Nab); cell-based and non-cell-based assay platforms, including bi-specific antibody drugs. She has acquired a highly diversified array of experience in pharmaceutical testing and has also developed a diversified skillset as a scientist, gaining valuable laboratory experience in both the GLP and GMP laboratory settings, while also participating and contributing during two FDA inspections, where she successfully completed all necessary requirements and experiments for her department during both inspections.

In October 2020, she quit her pharmaceutical career to switch over to Naturopathic Healing.

Pharmaceutical Work Experience:

2015-2018: Bioanalytical Scientist
Janssen Pharmaceutical R&D - Johnson & Johnson: Oncology & Immune Response Therapies in Biologics

2018-2019: Senior Chemist
AstraZeneca Manufacturing Global Operations: Quality Control Analytical Testing Experimentation

2019-2020: Laboratory Investigations Scientist
WuXi AppTec Advanced Therapies: Gene, Cell, & DNA Therapies - R&D and Finished Products - Quality Assurance

Education:

Mount St. Mary's University
Bachelor of Science (B.S.), Chemistry
2007-2011

Mount St. Mary's University
Master of Business Administration (M.B.A.), Finance
2011-2013

Six Sigma Yellow Belt
March 2019

Zinglepathy Rx was created by C.J. Zingle in October 2021. She had a vision of creating a one-stop online store where you could find health and wellness information as well as all the products relating to finding real health cures and soulutions.

Her passion and vision stem from her own health journey of trying to find answers from many different doctors and being told to "just deal with it" and that "there are no 'known' cures for your disease." After many years of wasting a ton of money and time, she stumbled upon (was guided to) a product called "Zeoboost", a brand of Zeolite powder. She began her journey using Zeoboost in July 2021 and saw immediate change in her health after 1 week of taking 6 teaspoons daily. Each week she noticed new and greater changes, and after 90 days, felt better than she had as a young kid. In 2013, she was diagnosed with Hashimotos (an autoimmune disease) after her health had gotten progressively worse, beginning around 2011. After doing much research on her own to find answers, she realized that her illness may have been caused by a vaccine injury in 2008, that she had gotten prior to being awake to the dangerous chemical ingredients in vaccines and their impact on our overall health. At the time, she was only 19 years old, and her primary care doctor had recommended to get the HPV vaccine "Gardasil", and being young and naïve, she agreed to get it and life began to change from there. She had played two Division 1 sports in college and then began suffering from many unbearable health symptoms such as chronic fatigue, psoriasis, and deep depression. She then learned there was a link, when she heard that her cousin (1 year older) had also started to develop symptoms of Lupus around the same time she had developed Hashimotos symptoms, and learned that her cousin had also gotten the Gardasil vaccine around the same time.

Our store offers natural herbal healing recommendations regarding any current health concerns/conditions in hopes of improving overall health around the world!

I myself have health conditions that doctors have not been able to help with and have found much relief through herbal healing, natural remedies and products. My experiences have made me want to help others in similar situations, because I know what it feels like to be hopeless, with no answers from modern medicine, and especially because I have gained so much knowledge of herbal medicine over the past few years in my own journey. Here at my store, you will find beneficial herbs and products, dosing, and how to take them for best results. I determine which herbs and products are best for you through intuitive practices AND medical research, to offer you the best recommendations and advice. I am an ex-R&D pharmacist, now turned FARMacist, who studies herbal medicine and soulutions, so I understand both sides of medicine and have a solid foundation in a wide variety of disease states.

Thank you for joining me on this journey!

You deserve to get your health back and live pain free!

Follow Me Here For More Updates:

Email: Rx@zinglepathy.com

Follow me on Truth Social & AnonUp for new insights and inspiration daily: @cjzingle

TikTok: @cjzingle

Instagram: @cjzingle

My Telegram Channel: https://t.me/xoanara

Personal Blog: Zinglepathy: Naturopathic Healing - https://www.zinglepathy.com/

My Online Store For Natural Remedies: https://form.jotform.com/Zinglepathy_Rx/detox-order-form

Made in the USA
Las Vegas, NV
12 January 2024

84257505R00070